BodyWisdom

A Note to the Reader
The material in this book is not intended to replace treatment by your doctor.
Its adoption and application is at the reader's discretion. Neither the authors nor the
publisher can be held responsible for any injury that may occur through following
instructions in this book.

First published in the United States in 1995 by
Charles E. Tuttle Company Inc. of Rutland, Vermont and Tokyo, Japan,
with editorial offices at 153 Milk Street, Boston, Massachusetts 02109.

Library of Congress Cataloging-in-Publication Data

Ruhnke, Amiyo.
    Body wisdom : simple massage and relaxation techniques for
busy people / by Amiyo Ruhnke and Anando Würzburger.
        p.   cm.
    ISBN 0-8048-3081-9
    1. Relaxation. 2. Exercise 3. Mind and body. 4. Meditation.
5. Massage. I. Würzburger, Anando II. Title.
RA785.R84   1995
613.7' 1–dc20   95-25026
                                                                    CIP

1   3   5   7   9   10   8   6   4   2

Designed by Amiyo Ruhnke
Photography by Sammy Hart
(except pages 4, 31, 42-43, 143, 153 by permission
of Osho Foundation International)
Illustrations by Russell Barnett

Colour Separation by Orange
Printed and bound in Great Britain by The Bath Press

Amiyo Ruhnke and
Anando Würzburger

Body**Wisdom**

An easy-to-use handbook of simple exercises
and self-massage techniques for busy people

Charles E. Tuttle Co., Inc.
Boston • Rutland, Vermont • Tokyo

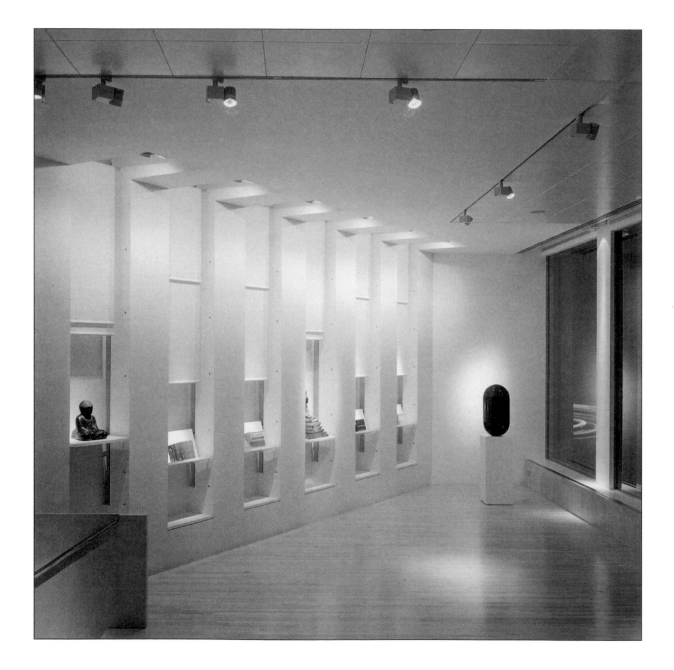

ACKNOWLEDGMENTS

THE DEVELOPMENT OF the concept for this book took place over a period of months in India, Germany and the U.K., and its production was undertaken by an international team representing those three countries, as well as Japan, and the United States. We worked hard, laughed a lot, and sometimes wondered what we had got ourselves into. Our deepest gratitude is to Osho, whose reverence for life, and light-hearted approach to its ups and downs, has inspired the project from start to finish.

In addition, we would like to acknowledge the following, without whose support and contribution the book would not have been possible:

Osho International Foundation, for permission to use Osho's words throughout the book.

Mukta and Samada, for making Osho International Gallery in London available as an informal photography studio, and for meeting the resulting disruptions to their work with good humour and grace.

Garjan and Anubuddha, for sharing their approach to bodywork with us.

Nishta for stress-relieving organisational skills.

Prabhu, for using part of his English holiday to help us get the first presentation materials together.

Sammy, for being in the moment, frame by frame, as he took the pictures, and Arunima, Gitama, Mukta, Samada, Sarito, Shinji and Rajen, for being relaxed and meditative enough to serve as models for the photographs.

Upavan, for not only opening doors and flagging down cabs, but doing a pretty good doodle when it's needed.

Jayesh, Sahajanand and Rajen for their ongoing support, encouragement and understanding.

Ian and the Orange Crew, for service above and far beyond the call of duty.

Sarito, for her invaluable contributions to both the form and content of the text, and Linda for all her editorial assistance.

Bob and the Apex typesetters, for their outstanding patience and professionalism.

Michael Alcock, Gordon Scott Wise and everyone at Boxtree for their trust and enthusiam for the book.

Amiyo Ruhnke and Anando Würzburger

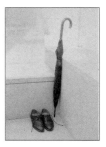

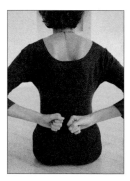

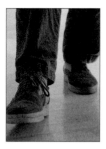

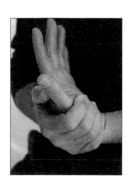

INTRODUCTION

OUR BODIES WERE beautifully designed for the purpose of hunting and gathering food, and for making the tools necessary to help us in that task. And, for most of human history, we have used our bodies exactly as they were designed to be used. But in the last century or so, the inventions of our imaginative and restless minds have brought us to the point where fewer and fewer of us have any opportunities to use our bodies very much at all.

In the course of our everyday lives, most of us spend most of our time sitting. We move from one place to another while sitting in automobiles and buses and trains. We sit at desks in front of computer screens and on couches in front of television sets. We turn on the tap when we need water, and we toss our dirty clothing into automatic washing machines. The only exercise most of us get in pursuit of our food is in totting bags from the car to the kitchen, and putting them away on the shelves.

As a result, we have lost most of the natural flexibility and aliveness of the body. Furthermore, we are so accustomed to our state that most of us don't even realize it until something goes so wrong that the body has to send an SOS in the form of pain. Because we spend so much time living on our backsides and in our heads, our ability to be sensitive to the body and receptive to its needs has been dulled. This insensitivity sets up a vicious circle: the less we move, the more insensitive we become to what the body needs and wants; the less we do for the body, the less energy we have available.

The less energy we have, the more we are inclined just to sit on our backsides and live in our heads!

BodyWisdom is a simple guide to gently reawakening the body's aliveness and flexibility. It's a celebration of the body's exquisite design, and an encouragement to the body to use its natural wisdom in telling us what it needs. It is an acknowledgment of the deep interdependence of body and mind, and a guide to helping the mind step aside from time to time, so the body can have its say. As you read, it should become obvious that that *BodyWisdom* is not really technique oriented, although there are plenty of techniques in its pages. It's not a collection of things to "do to" your body – this is important. The techniques and exercises are just devices, really, ways to bring you more together in body, mind and spirit.

Finally, it's an introduction to meditation, using the body as the simplest and most natural door to the relaxation and enjoyment meditation can bring. We know you don't have time to meditate, or time to look after the needs of your body – and we've taken that into account. Most of the exercises are designed to fit easily and naturally into your activities from day to day. Read through the book first, and take note of what exercises and techniques appeal to you and seem to fit with your needs. Then start trying them out, and continue with the ones you like. Once you get off your backside and out of your head, you'll be better able to hear the whispers of your own body's wisdom, and taking care of yourself will come more naturally.

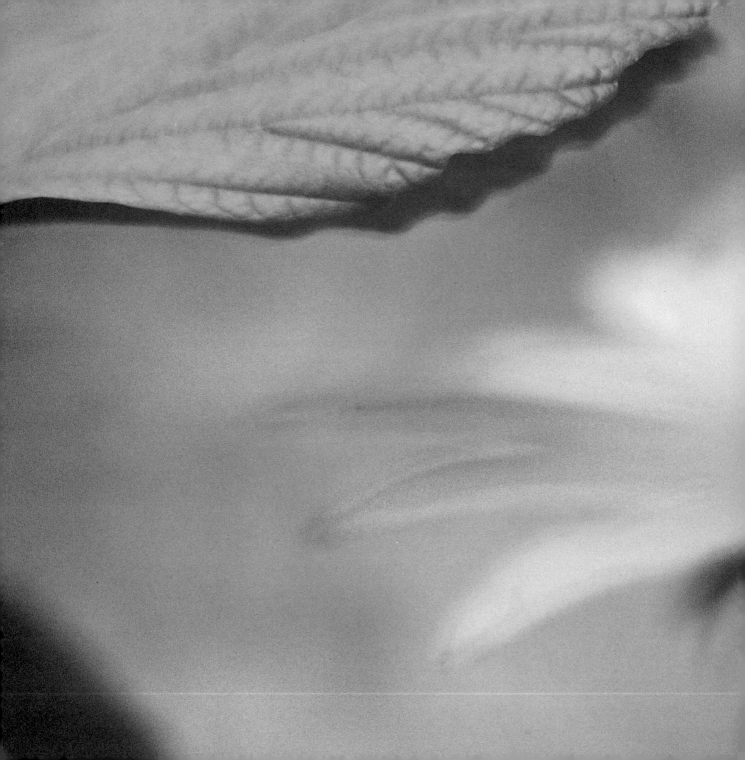

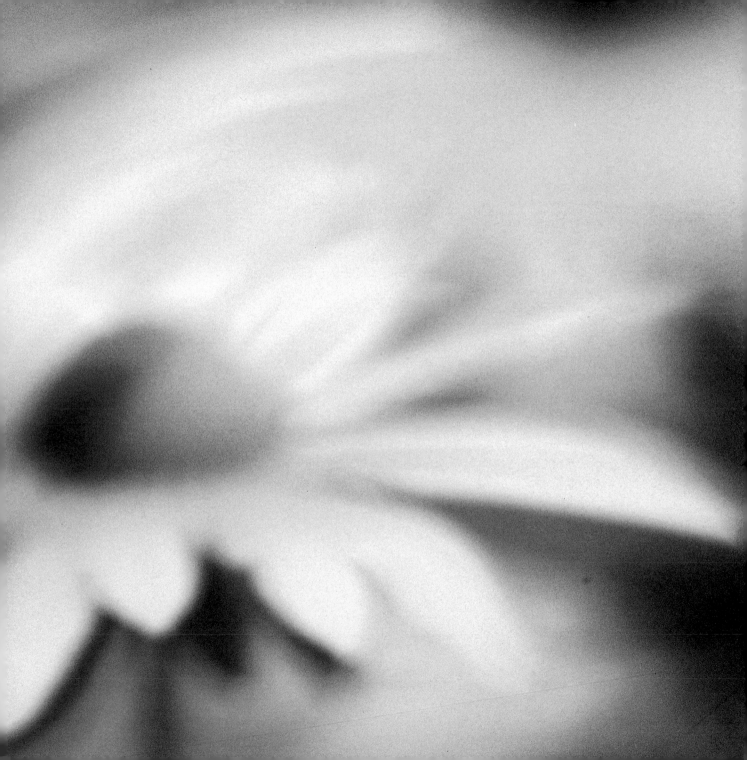

Body Basics
Beneath the Skin: A Guide to What's What, and Where

Most of us, unless we have been trained in one of the healing professions, have only the vaguest notion of what we look like underneath the skin. Nature generally manages things in such a way that we don't need to know, in fact. Our bodies go on taking nourishment and distributing it where it's needed, eliminating waste and harmful bacteria, sending and receiving messages and carrying out millions of other complex tasks without any conscious help from us at all.

For the most part, this is as it should be. The conscious mind can be a real mischief-maker when it is allowed to interfere in matters that are outside its proper domain — like bringing logic into a love affair, or trying to measure beauty in a scientific laboratory. If we let our minds get involved in digesting our lunch, for example, we're likely to end up with indigestion! But if the power of the mind is joined with a little bit of awareness it can be a tremendous help in staying in tune with our body's needs and responding to

those needs in a creative and healing way.

The pictures on the opposite page is intended to help you get acquainted with what's what and where beneath your skin. So that the next time you feel that slightly burning ache in your lower back you can consider the possibility that your kidneys are suffering and you need to drink more water. Or, that the dull ache in your right side might be your liver trying to tell you to clean up your act. It's also so that when you get to the "meridian stretches" later on in the book, which help to tone and strengthen the organs of the body, your mind will be able to help the process with a reasonably accurate image of each organ and where it is.

Not to think about it too much, not to demystify its miraculous workings, or to drag the wonder of it into the scientific lab. But just to get acquainted with it, to be a little more intelligent about it, to make friends with it and allow it to make friends with you.

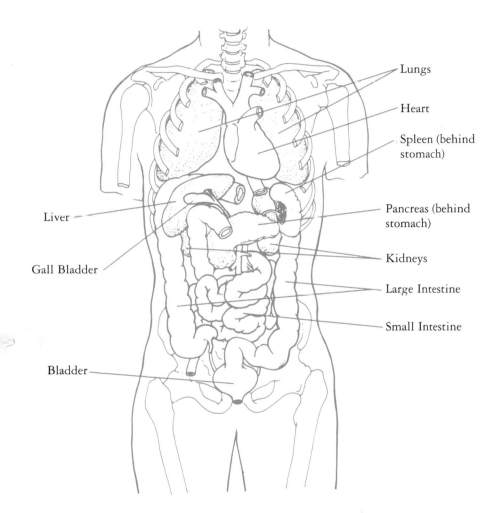

Lungs

Heart

Spleen (behind stomach)

Pancreas (behind stomach)

Kidneys

Large Intestine

Small Intestine

Liver

Gall Bladder

Bladder

...And the body is a miracle; it is tremendously beautiful, tremendously complex. There is no other thing so complex, so subtle as the body. You don't know anything about it. You have only looked at it in the mirror. You have never looked at it from the within; otherwise it is a universe in itself. That's what the mystics have always been saying: that the body is a miniature universe. If you see it from the inside, it is so vast — millions and millions of cells, and each cell alive with its own life, and each cell functioning in such an intelligent manner that it seems almost incredible, impossible, unbelievable.[2]

The Miniature You in Your Ear

MOST PEOPLE BY now have heard of the ancient Chinese healing system of acupuncture, if they have not actually experienced it themselves. Less common is to have a basic understanding of the principles underlying it, and why it works.

Western medicine for centuries has developed in the direction of treating the body as a collection of separate parts. If the tonsils tend to get regularly inflamed, they can be taken out. If somebody has "heart trouble" or "kidney trouble" there are drugs available to treat these specific organs. If we have an infection we treat it with antibiotics, if we have a vitamin deficiency we take tablets to correct it.

The oriental systems of medicine such as acupuncture and shiatsu have a very different view of things. They see the body as one organic whole, whose health depends on an unobstructed and balanced flow of "chi" or vital energy. Finely detailed maps of the channels in which this energy flows – known as "meridians" – help to guide the oriental healing practitioner in locating areas where the flow might be obstructed. At various points along the meridians, either finger pressure or needles can be applied to stimulate and rebalance the flow. The same points can also be used to interrupt the flow of energy if the situation demands it. That's why, for example, acupuncture can be used as an anesthetic.

There are many excellent books on the subject of oriental healing, and we can offer only the briefest glimpse into this complex subject here. On this page, and the pages which follow, are a few of the maps which show the wondrous harmonies built into our bodies. Just having a look at them can give you a whole new perspective on the "body basics" – and help you to understand some of the exercises presented later on in the book.

CHINESE MEDICINE HAS discovered that there are acupuncture points on the ear which correspond to those on the body as a whole, as this picture shows. So think twice before you have that new hole punched in your ear for yet another earring!! Seriously, though – this illustration makes it clear why a good ear massage (see page 45) first thing in the morning, or at a low point in the day, can make you feel fresher and more alive all over.

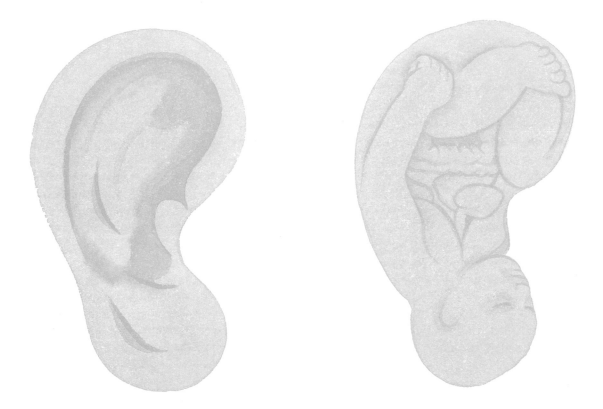

It's all in the Feet: Who's Who Inside Your Shoes

THERE IS A story about Mulla Nasruddin, the wise fool of the Sufis, who was in the habit of complaining bitterly about his aching feet and the fact that his shoes were pinching him. Finally, a friend took pity on him and offered to buy Nasruddin a new pair of shoes. He accepted the offer and they went together to a fine shop in the market, where Nasruddin tried on several pairs before finding one that suited him. "This style is good," he said to the shop-keeper. "Now bring me a pair one size smaller than this."

"But that will be too small," the shopkeeper protested. "The shoes will pinch your feet and cause them to ache all day long."
"I know, I know," replied Nasruddin. "But when they are too tight, it is such a great joy to take them off – in fact my life is so hard, and the only pleasure I have the whole day long is when I finally get home from work and take off my shoes."

The map on this page suggests that Nasruddin was being more foolish than wise in this particular instance. His shoes were pinching not only his feet but all the vital organs in body! No wonder his life was so hard....

All the organs in the body are represented in the soles of the feet, providing us with a convenient way to treat ourselves to a relaxing and revitalizing massage. Try it, using oil or cream to help you press deeply with your fingers, and experiment with how the feet can bend and stretch. Notice what points on your feet feel sore or tender. It could be that the organ associated with that spot needs some loving attention from you right now.

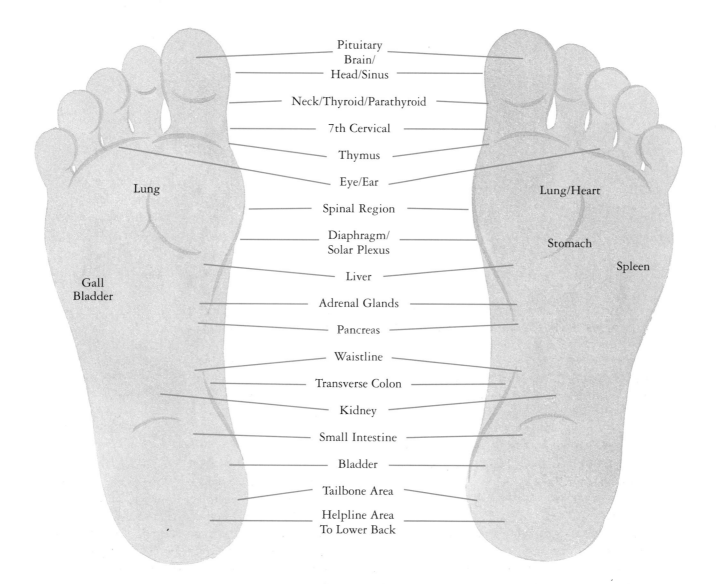

Pituitary

Brain/
Head/Sinus

Neck/Thyroid/Parathyroid

7th Cervical

Thymus

Eye/Ear

Lung

Lung/Heart

Spinal Region

Diaphragm/
Solar Plexus

Stomach

Liver

Spleen

Gall
Bladder

Adrenal Glands

Pancreas

Waistline

Transverse Colon

Kidney

Small Intestine

Bladder

Tailbone Area

Helpline Area
To Lower Back

Breath and the Rhythm of Life

THROUGHOUT THE BOOK we will be reminding you to be aware of your breath, to make sure you aren't holding it, or to coordinate the movements of an exercise with the inhalation or exhalation of breath. In India, the word for breath and vitality is the same, *prana*. Here is just a brief introduction to the importance of the breath, and a meditation you can try in order to understand its role in your health and wellbeing. It is excerpted from a talk by Osho.

Sit silently; listen to all that is happening all around, and relax; accept, relax – and suddenly you will feel immense energy arising in you. That energy will be felt first as a deepening of your breath. Ordinarily your breath is very shallow and sometimes if you try to have deep breaths, if you start doing *pranayam* (yoga breathing exercises) you start forcing something, you make an effort. That effort is not needed. You simply accept life, relax, and suddenly you will see that your breath is going deeper than ever. Relax more and the breath goes deeper in you. It becomes slow, rhythmic, and you can almost enjoy it; it gives a certain delight. Then you will become aware that breath is the bridge between you and the whole.

Just watch. Don't do anything. And when I say watch, don't *try* to watch, otherwise you will become tense again, and you will start concentrating on the breath. Simply relax, remain relaxed, loose, and look...because what else can you do? You are there, nothing to be done, everything accepted, nothing to be denied, rejected, no struggle, no fight, no conflict, breathing going deep – what can you do? You simply watch. Remember, simply watch. Don't make an effort to watch. This is what Buddha has called *vipassana* – the watching of the breath, awareness of the breath – or *satipatthana* – remembering, being alert of the life energy that moves in breath. Don't try to take deep breaths, don't try to inhale or exhale, don't do anything. You simply relax and let the breathing be natural – going on its own, coming on its own – and many things will become available to you.

The first thing will be that breathing can be taken in two ways because it is a bridge. One part of it is joined with you, another part is joined with existence. So it can be understood in two ways. You can take it as a voluntary thing. If you want to inhale deeply, you can inhale deeply; if you want to exhale deeply, you can exhale deeply. You can do something about it. One part is joined with you. But if you don't do anything, then too it continues. No need for you to do anything and it continues. It is non-voluntary also.

The other part is joined with existence itself. You can think of it as if you are taking it in, you are breathing it, or you can think in just the opposite way – that it is breathing you. And the other way has to be understood because that will lead you into deep relaxation. It is not that you are breathing, but existence is breathing you. It is a change of gestalt, and it happens on its own. If you go on relaxing, accepting everything, relaxing into yourself, by and by, suddenly, you become aware that you are not taking these breaths – they are coming and going on their own. And so gracefully. With such dignity. With such rhythm. With such harmonious rhythm. Who is doing it? Existence is breathing you. It comes into you, goes out of you. Each moment it rejuvenates you, each moment it makes you alive again and again and again.[3] *"*

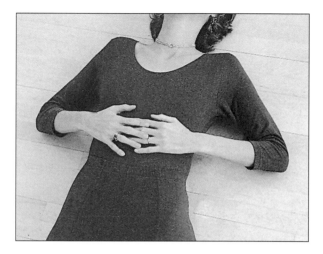

THE EXERCISE ILLUSTRATED ON THIS PAGE IS AS FOLLOWS:

Find a place in your body where you feel comfortable, at home, at ease. Put both your hands on that part of your body and imagine your breath going into that place and being nourished and strengthened there. When you are quite settled in this place, notice where in your body you are feeling tense. Take one hand and put it on the tense place.

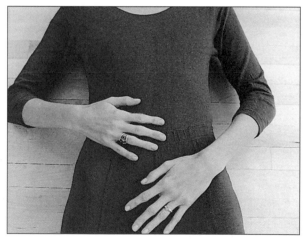

As you inhale, imagine the breath entering into the place where you are comfortable, gathering all that comfort and ease. As you exhale, imagine the breath leaving the body through the place where you are feeling tense, allowing the tension to dissolve with the outgoing breath. Continue as long as it feels good to do so, allowing the breath to remain relaxed and natural.

Body Safari

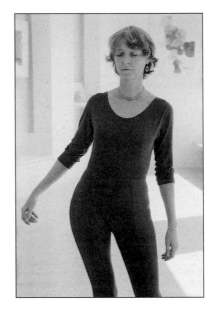

ONE UNFORTUNATE BY-product of the sedentary life most of us lead these days is that the moving parts of our bodies begin to lose their natural flexibility. It's as if the joints get rusty, and the muscles surrounding them get set in certain patterns. That can block the free and natural flow of energy in our bodies, which in turn makes us feel less like moving, which means we lose even more flexibility, and so on it goes.

The pictures on this page are just hints to help you get started on your own "body safari," an expedition to explore all the ways your body can move. We suggest you start with the feet: plant them on the floor about as far apart as the width of your shoulders, and let yourself settle until you feel balanced and steady. There's no particular goal here, no "right" way to do it, no need to have an idea of where you're going and no reason to

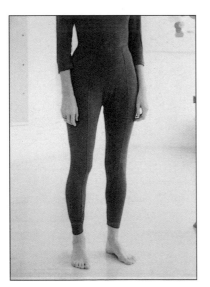

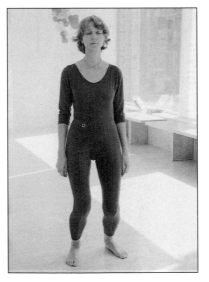

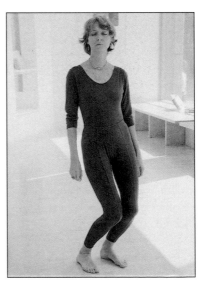

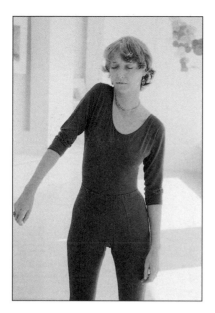

push. It's just a playful exploration, letting your body show you what it can do.

Prepare to begin by closing your eyes, letting your jaw drop open so your face is relaxed. Take a few moments to pay attention to your breathing, and then as you inhale imagine that the breath is going to all the joints in your body, lubricating them just like you'd use an oil can on a squeaky door. Now you're ready to begin experimenting with all the ways your body can move. If the movements happen in little jerks, that's just tension stored there. As you go on, these movements will start to smoothe out, so don't worry about it.... Ready?

While you are standing there, imagine that you are growing roots into the floor, into the earth. This will help you feel secure and grounded for the rest of the exploration. Now move upward, from the toes through the bones of the foot, to the ankles. Allow the ankles to open, to hold you in a relaxed way as you experiment with moving in small circles, then larger circles,

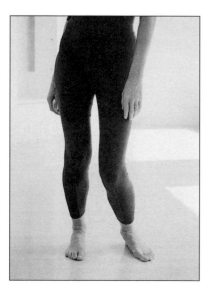
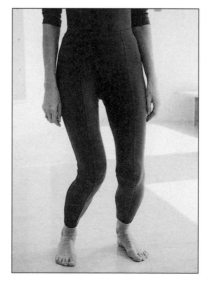
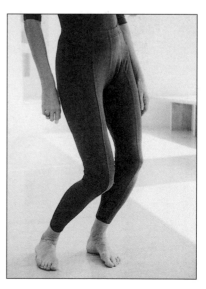

letting the ankles show you how they can support you and yet be fluid and flexible. Move up to the knees, and explore how they can move forward and back, from side to side, and around in circles.

Work your way up from the ground, and stay in touch with how your body is feeling. Don't push it past the point where it feels like a pleasant stretch, and experiment with both larger movements and smaller ones, watching as you go. The point is to feel from the inside how your joints can move, to explore the space in there and to allow it to open up and relax, to become more flexible. Try being a piece of seaweed on the bottom of the ocean, with your roots planted on the ocean floor and your tendrils being washed this way and that by the currents in the water. Don't be afraid to make a fool of yourself — nobody's watching! And remember to breathe....

Be a jellyfish, and feel what it's like to float. Be a belly dancer in slow motion, and move your pelvis accordingly. Remember the hula hoop? Imagine you have one, but there's no need to go fast to keep it falling to the

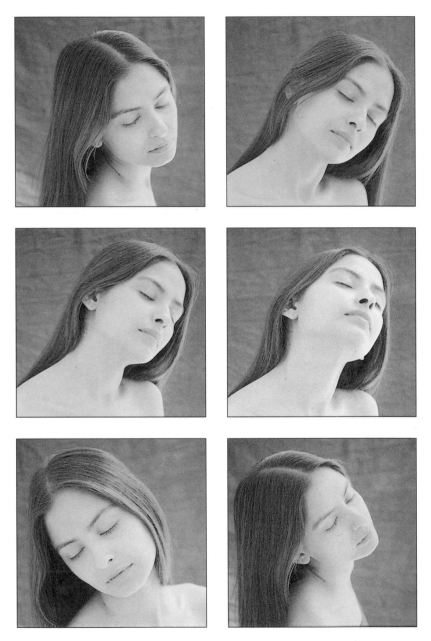

floor. Explore the movements you can make with your hands, finger by finger and then with the wrists... see how graceful your hands can be?

When you get to your shoulders, experiment with letting them move in circles, smaller and then larger, one shoulder at a time and then both together. Are you still breathing? Is the movement a little bit jerky, or smooth? Does it change depending on the size of the circle you're making? Close your eyes and travel inside, right inside your right shoulder. Make the circle so subtle, so small that you're sure it can't be seen from the outside, even though you can feel it from the inside. Now do the same with the left shoulder.

When you're done, take a deep breath, and let it out slowly, watching it as it goes.

The Body Safari is something you can come back to as often as you like, whenever you have a little time between this and that in your schedule. Each time you come back to it, see if anything has changed, feels easier, is more fun to do.

Before we leave the Body Safari behind, there's one last bit we haven't covered. The neck. For many of us, it's where the most tension collects in our bodies – especially those of us who work at a desk all day long. The gentle movements shown on the opposite page can be done many times throughout the day, and will go a long way towards relaxing not only the neck and shoulders, but your whole body. You can do them while sitting at the desk, stuck in a traffic jam, or when you're sitting in front of the television. Our model has her eyes closed, which definitely adds another dimension to the exercises, but it's not strictly necessary.

TRY IT LIKE THIS AT FIRST, AND THEN MAKE UP YOUR OWN VARIATIONS:

1 Turn your head slowly to one side as far as it will comfortably go, keeping the chin level and the shoulders relaxed. Then return to the centre, and repeat the movement two more times. Now turn to the opposite side and back to the centre, three times.

2 Let your head move gently forward, until you feel a pull of the muscles at the back of your neck. Return to an upright position, and repeat the movement two more times. Go slowly, allow yourself to feel the movement and what it does to the muscles of the neck as you go.

3 Let your head move gently backward in the same way, and then return to an upright position three times, slowly and gently.

4 Now experiment with diagonal movements of the head in the same way. This is quite an uncommon movement, and may feel a little awkward at first. Take it easy, so you don't strain the neck muscles. It might help to imagine a compass, and you are moving your head northwest and then southeast, northeast and then southwest.

5 Finish up with a rolling circular movement of the head, slowly and gently so you don't strain the muscles of the neck. Make a full circle in one direction, then reverse and go in the other direction.

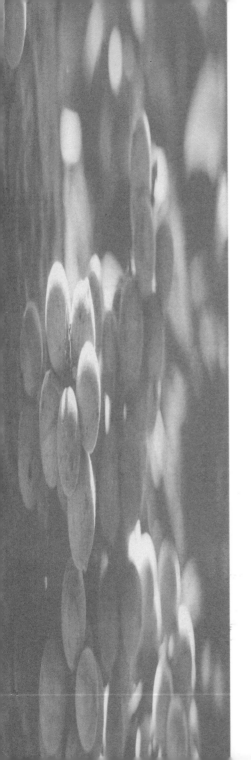

"The body is your earth; you are rooted in the body. Your consciousness is like a tree in the body. Your thoughts are like fruits. Your meditations are like flowers. But you are rooted in the body; the body supports it. The body supports everything that you are doing. You love; the body supports. You hate; the body supports. You want to kill somebody; the body supports. You want to protect somebody; the body supports. In compassion, in love, in anger, in hate – in every way – the body supports you. You are rooted in the body; you are nourished by the body. Even when you start realizing who you are, the body supports you. Don't kill the body. Don't be a masochist, don't torture it. It is your friend; it is not your enemy. Listen to its language, decode its language, and by and by, as you enter into the book of the body and you turn its pages, you will become aware of the whole mystery of life. Condensed, it is in your body. Magnified a millionfold, it is all over the world. But condensed in a small formula, it is there present in your body. Decode it there first."[4]

Getting It Together

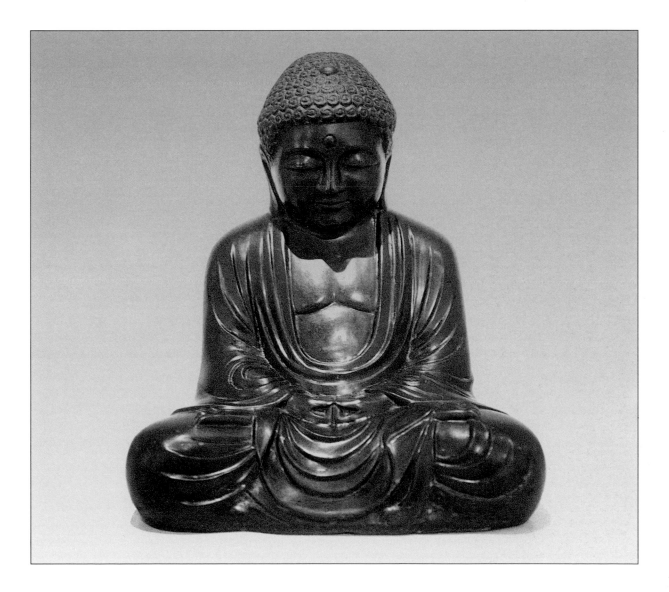

BEFORE WE GO on to the specific exercises contained in the rest of the book, a few more things need to be said. We're going to let Osho do a lot of the talking here, for a couple of reasons. The first is because he says it so beautifully, and the second is because he has done a tremendous amount of work with people in helping them to both understand and experience the integration of body, mind and spirit. That integration, that harmony, is what makes us feel truly healthy and whole. It's not about looking like this year's supermodel, or next year's action hero. It's about discovering the unique fingerprint of our own BodyWisdom, so we can consciously nourish it and help it to grow. The process begins, as Osho explains below, by dropping all our ideas about how we "should" be.

The Body You Have...

" If you have a certain idea about how the body should be, you will be in misery. The body is as it should be. If you have some idea you will be in misery, so drop that idea.

This is the body you have; this is the body god has given to you. Use it... enjoy it! And if you start loving it, you will find it is changing, because if a person loves his body he starts taking care, and care implies everything. Then you don't stuff it with unnecessary food, because you care. Then you don't starve it, because you care. You listen to its demands, you listen to its hints – what it wants, when it wants. When you care, when you love, you become attuned to the body, and the body automatically becomes okay. If you don't like the body, that will create the problem, because then by and by you will become indifferent to the body, negligent of the body, because who cares about the enemy? You will not look at it; you will avoid it. You will stop listening to its messages, and then you will hate it more – and you are creating the whole problem!

The body never creates any problem; it is the mind that creates problems. Now, this is an idea of the mind. No animal suffers from any idea about the body, no animal – not even the hippopotamus! Nobody suffers, they are perfectly happy because no mind is there to create an idea; otherwise the hippopotamus will think 'Why am I like this?'

There is no problem in it, just drop the ideal. Love your body – this is your body, this is a gift from god. You have to enjoy it and you have to take care of it. When you take care, you exercise, you eat, you sleep. You take every care because this is your instrument, just like your car that you clean, that you listen to, to every hum – to know whether something is going wrong. You take care even if a scratch comes on the body. Just take care of the body and it will be perfectly beautiful – it is! It is such a beautiful mechanism, and so complex, and yet working so efficiently that for 70 years it goes on functioning. Whether you are asleep or awake, aware or unaware, it goes on functioning, and the functioning is so silent. Even without your caring it goes on functioning; it goes on doing service to you. One should be grateful to the body.

Just change your attitude and you will see that within six months your body has changed its form. It is almost like when you fall in love with a woman and you see: she immediately becomes beautiful. She may not have cared about her body up to this moment but when a man falls in love with her, she starts taking care. She stands before the mirror for hours... because somebody loves her! The same happens: you love your body and you will see that your body has started changing. It is loved, it is taken care of, it is needed. It is a very delicate mechanism – people use it very crudely, violently. Just change your attitude and see![5] "

Acceptance of where we are is the first step in nourishing our own BodyWisdom, but it's by no means the whole journey. Once we have put aside our notions of how we should be, we are free to simply observe how we are, in a relaxed way, without any judgment or condemnation. The easiest place to begin this watching, or this observation

Use it! Enjoy it!

– which is really the essence of all meditation – is in the activities of the body. Are you getting worried that by watching, rather than "getting lost" in what you're doing, you'll become so detached and other-worldly that you won't have any fun anymore? Relax! Just experiment with it, and see.... Here are a few words of wisdom to take with you on the journey.

" Total relaxation is the ultimate. That's the moment when one becomes a buddha. That is the moment of realization, enlightenment, christ-consciousness. You cannot be totally relaxed right now. At the innermost core a tension will persist.

But start relaxing. Start from the circumference – that's where we are, and we can start only from where we are. Relax the circumference of your being – relax your body, relax your behavior, relax your acts. Walk in a relaxed way, eat in a relaxed way, talk, listen in a relaxed way. Slow down every process. Don't be in a hurry and don't be in haste. Move as if all eternity is available to you – in fact, it is available to you. We are here from the beginning and we are going to be here to the very end, if there is a beginning and there is an end. In fact, there is no beginning and no end. We have always been here and we will be here always. Forms go on changing, but not the substance; garments go on changing, but not the soul.

Tension means hurry, fear, doubt. Tension means a constant effort to protect, to be secure, to be safe. Tension means preparing for the tomorrow now, or for the afterlife — afraid tomorrow you will not be able to face the reality, so be prepared. Tension means the past that you have not lived really but only somehow by passed; it hangs, it is a hangover, it surrounds you.

Remember one very fundamental thing about life: any experience that has not been lived will hang around you, will persist; "Finish me! Live me! Complete me!" There is an intrinsic quality in every experience that it tends and wants to be finished, completed. Once completed, it evaporates; incomplete, it persists, it tortures you, it haunts you, it attracts your attention. It says, "What are you going to do about me? I am still incomplete – fulfil me!"
Your whole past hangs around you with nothing completed — because nothing has been lived really, everything somehow by passed, partially lived, only so-so, in a lukewarm way. There has been no intensity, no passion. You have been moving like a somnambulist, a sleepwalker. So that past hangs, and the future creates fear. And between the past and the future is crushed your present, the only reality.

You will have to relax from the circumference. The first step in relaxing is the body. Remember as many times as possible to look in the body, whether you are carrying some tension in the body somewhere — at the neck, in the head, in the legs. Relax it consciously. Just go to that part of the body, and persuade that part, say to it lovingly "Relax!"
And you will be surprised that if you approach any part of your body, it listens, it follows you – it is your body! With closed eyes, go inside the body from the toes to the head searching for any place where there is a tension. And then talk to that part as you talk to a friend; let there be a dialogue between you and your body. Tell it to relax, and tell it, "There is nothing to fear. Don't be afraid. I am here to take care – you can relax." Slowly slowly, you will learn the knack of it. Then the body becomes relaxed.

Start from the Body...

Then take another step, a little deeper; tell the mind to relax. And if the body listens, mind also listens, but you cannot start with the mind — you have to start from the beginning. You cannot start from the middle. Many people start with the mind and they fail; they fail because they start from a wrong place. Everything should be done in the right order.

If you become capable of relaxing the body voluntarily, then you will be able to help your mind relax voluntarily. Mind is a more complex phenomenon. Once you have become confident that the body listens to you, you will have a new trust in yourself. Now even the mind can listen to you. It will take a little longer with the mind, but it happens.

When the mind is relaxed, then start relaxing your heart, the world of your feelings, emotions – which is even more complex, more subtle. But now you will be moving with trust, with great trust in yourself. Now you will know it is possible. If it is possible with the body and possible with the mind, it is possible with the

...And Then Go Deeper

heart too. And then only, when you have gone through these three steps, can you take the fourth. Now you can go to the innermost core of your being, which is beyond body, mind, heart: the very center of your existence. And you will be able to relax it too.

And that relaxation certainly brings the greatest joy possible, the ultimate in ecstasy, acceptance. You will be full of bliss and rejoicing. Your life will have the quality of dance to it.

The whole of existence is dancing, except man. The whole of existence is in a very relaxed movement; movement there is, certainly, but it is utterly relaxed. Trees are growing and birds are chirping and rivers are flowing, stars are moving: everything is going in a very relaxed way. No hurry, no haste, no worry, and no waste. Except man. Man has fallen a victim of his mind.

Man can rise above gods and fall below animals. Man has a great spectrum. From the lowest to the highest, man is a ladder.

Start from the body, and then go, slowly slowly, deeper. And don't start with anything else unless you have first solved the primary. If your body is tense, don't start with the mind. Wait. Work on the body. And just small things are of immense help.

You walk at a certain pace; that has become habitual, automatic. Now try to walk slowly. Buddha used to say to his disciples, "Walk very slowly, and take each step very consciously." If you take each step very consciously, you are bound to walk slowly. If you are running, hurrying, you will forget to remember. Hence Buddha walks very slowly.

Just try walking very slowly, and you will be surprised – a new quality of awareness starts happening in the body. Eat slowly, and you will be surprised – there is great relaxation. Do everything slowly ... just to change the old pattern, just to come out of old habits.

Total Relaxation is Paradise

First the body has to become utterly relaxed, like a small child, then only start with the mind. Move scientifically: first the simplest, then the complex, then the more complex. And only then can you relax at the ultimate core....

Relaxation is one of the most complex phenomena – very rich, multidimensional. All these things are part of it: let-go, trust, surrender, love, acceptance, going with the flow, union with existence, egolessness, ecstasy. All these are part of it, and all these start happening if you learn the ways of relaxation.

Your so-called religions have made you very tense, because they have created guilt in you. My effort is to help you get rid of all guilt and all fear. I would like to tell you: there is no hell and no heaven. So don't be afraid of hell and don't be greedy for heaven. All that exists is this moment. You can make this moment a hell or a heaven – that certainly is possible – but there is no heaven or hell somewhere else. Hell is when you are all tense, and heaven is when you are all relaxed. Total relaxation is paradise.[6] "

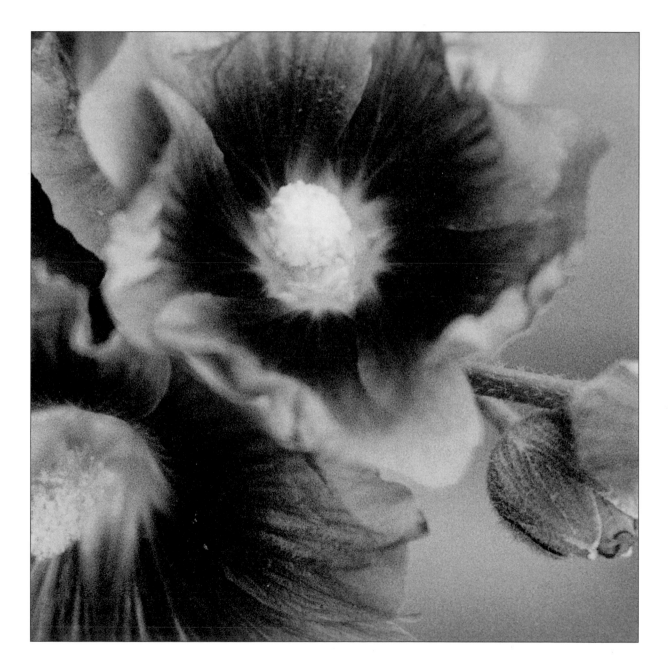

Finding Your Roots, Spreading Your Wings

HAVE YOU EVER seen one of those little dolls — or sometimes they come as a kind of inflatable "punching bag" for children — which is weighted on the bottom, so no matter which way you try to knock it down, it always comes back to stand upright again? Legend has it that these dolls were invented in Japan as a tribute to the great Zen master Bodhidharma. He was so "grounded, " so "centred" that it was impossible to knock him off balance. The East has developed a variety of material arts and yoga to help people in reaching this state of being grounded, or centred. And our own language in the West reflects a kind of native wisdom about such things — we describe somebody as one who "has her feet on the ground," or, conversely, being "easily knocked off centre."

Just as we start with the body in learning to become more aware, more healthy and whole, so we start with where our bodies meet the earth in reconnecting with our BodyWisdom. If we're going to spread our branches into the sky, we have to make sure our roots are strong enough to support us in that journey to meet the stars.

> Every person moves in a different way, walks in a different way. If a Buddha walks he is tremendously grounded. His legs are almost like roots of a tree. He is in deep contact with the earth. He is nourished by the earth, the earth is nourished by him. There is a continuous transfer of energy. Ordinary people are uprooted trees. They walk as if they are uprooted; they don't have roots in the earth, they are not grounded. You try sometimes. Just stand with naked feet on the earth or on the sand on a beach and just feel that your legs are like roots and that they are reaching deep into the earth. And start swaying with the wind like a tree. Forget that you are a man, think of yourself as a tree, and soon you will see something transpiring between you and the earth. It may take a little time because you have forgotten the language but one day you will see something is transpiring. Something is given by the earth to the feet and you are also returning, responding. And the day it happens you will start walking in a totally new way — rooted, solid, not fragile, not sad, more alive, full of energy. You will be less tired and your footsteps will have a different quality.[7]

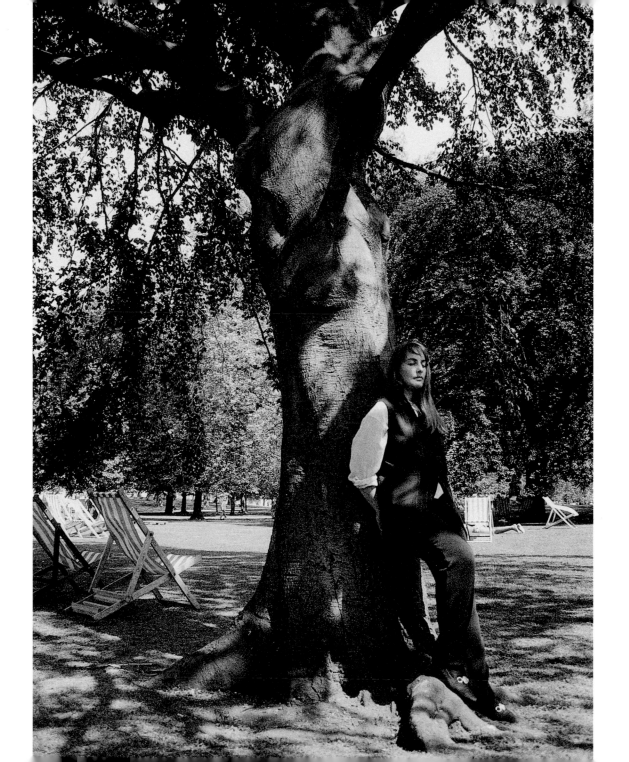

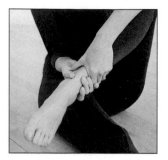

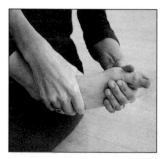

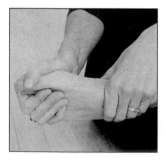

Getting Your Feet on the Ground

THE EXERCISE ROUTINE pictured on these pages is both a treat for your feet and a tangible experience of what it feels like to "get your feet on the ground." You'll feel the difference right away, and if you do it regularly you'll feel the benefit in better circulation in the legs, and a better sense of balance and "grounding" — that mysterious bodymind feeling of being yourself, spontaneous, unshakeable, and free to move in any direction.

Start by standing and just closing your eyes for a moment, feeling your feet on the ground. The following steps can be done sitting on floor if you are very flexible and accustomed to sitting cross-legged. If sitting on the floor causes pain or makes it difficult to do the steps of the exercise, then it is perfectly fine to sit in a chair or on the side of your bed. You can use a cream or oil if you like, to make the whole process a little more sensuous. The first time, do all the steps described on one foot before moving to the other: this will help you experience quite clearly the effects of the technique. It goes like this:

1 Grasp the ankle in both hands. Let the foot be limp and loose, and shake it vigorously for one or two minutes, as long as you can without tiring yourself. Be aware not to tense your shoulders, and just let the foot flop around like an old dust mop.

2/3 Holding the foot with one hand, grasp the toes and ball of the foot with the other hand and rotate it, first in one direction, and then in the other. Do all the work with your hands, don't let the foot get involved in this motion. Experiment with figure of eights, and see whether the foot becomes more flexible as you continue the rotations. Don't be worried about getting it just right, the idea is to open up space and relaxation there in the toes and the ball of the foot.

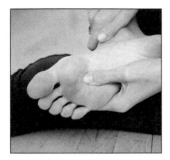

4 This is an opportunity to massage the kidney point on the bottom of the foot, the "bubbling spring" of Chinese medicine which connects you with the energy of the earth and brings its life and vitality into the body through your feet. If it feels very tender, spend a little extra time there, gently helping it to loosen up and relax.

5 Now interlock the toes with the fingers of the opposite hand. It may be difficult at first — most people, when they start, can only manage to get the tips of the fingers comfortably between the toes. But it won't be long before you'll find yourself being able to do what our model is doing in photo number 5. Keeping the fingers and toes interlocked, again move the foot in a circular motion, first one way and then the other, loosening and opening the area on the top of the foot where all those bones and tendons come to meet the base of the toes.

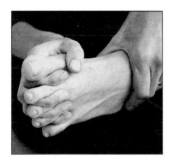

6 As you would cradle a baby, pick up the lower part of the leg with the knee in one elbow and the foot in the other, and rock it gently back and forth. This is to loosen and open up the hip joint. If you find it too hard at first to adopt the position shown here, you can sit in a chair, and cross your leg "macho style," with the ankle resting on the knee of the opposite leg. Then you can rock the crossed leg gently back and forth using your hands. Now, stand up again and feel the difference! Repeat the process for the other leg.

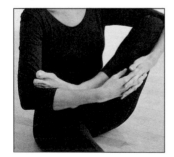

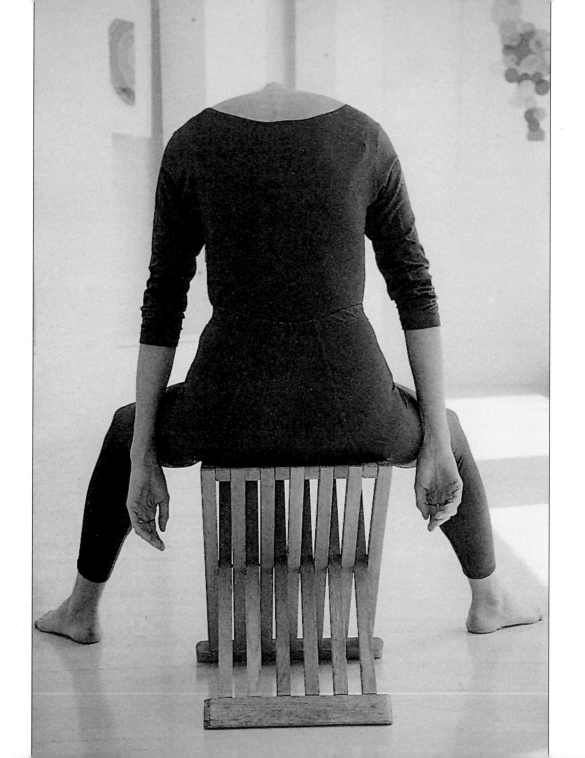

Easy is Right: Following the Movement from Within

IN ANCIENT JAPAN, if you asked somebody where his "thinking" was located, he would point to his belly. The Native Americans would point to the heart. Does it seem like an absurd idea, that we should think from the belly, or from the heart?

In fact, as we have mentioned earlier, the head is quite useful if it doesn't interfere in activities that are really none of its business. But it's rare these days to find anybody who would point to the heart or to the belly as the place that drives most of their activities in life. Most of us do "head work" and as a result our heads have become so overdeveloped that they have taken over far more than their share of our lives.

This last part of *Getting It Together* is about developing the capacity to be "headless." As that capacity grows in you, it will do two things: One: it will help you to get more benefit from the exercises that follow, because it will enhance your capacity to "feel" from the inside what is happening, what your body enjoys and needs. Two: it will help you to dissolve old patterns that your head has set up, patterns that contribute to making you tense and tired. As you become "headless" whether you find yourself dropping into your heart or into your belly depends on you, and your unique individuality. Here, Osho is answering questions from people who want to know how to move more into the heart. But the techniques he suggests can equally apply to those who feel most grounded and at ease when they are centered in the belly.

" Try it as a meditation. It is one of the most beautiful tantra meditations. Walk, and think that the head is no longer there – just the body. Sit, and think that the head is no longer there – just the body. Continuously remember that the head is not there. Visualize yourself without the head. Have a picture of yourself enlarged – without the head. Look at it. Let your mirror be lowered in the bathroom so when you look into it, you cannot see your head – just the body.

A few days of remembrance, and you will feel such weightlessness happening to you, such tremendous silence, because it is the head that is the problem. If you can conceive of yourself as headless.... And that can be conceived, there is no trouble in it. Then more and more, you'll be centered near the heart.[8]

" Whenever you deeply feel, you are headless. In that moment there is no head; there cannot be. The heart becomes your whole being – as if the head has disappeared. In feeling, the centre of being is the heart. While you are thinking, the centre of being is the head. But thinking proved very useful for survival, so we have stopped everything else. All other dimensions of our being have been stopped and closed. We are just heads, and the body is just a situation for the head to exist. We go on thinking; even about feelings we go on thinking. So try to feel. You will have to work on it, because that capacity, that quality, has remained retarded. You must do something to re-open that possibility.

You look at a flower and immediately you say it is beautiful. Ponder over the fact, linger over the fact. Don't give a hurried judgement. Wait – and then see whether it is just from the head that you have said it is beautiful, or whether you have felt it. Is it just a routine thing, because you know a rose is beautiful, supposed to be beautiful? People say it is beautiful, and you have also said many times that it is beautiful.

The moment you see the rose, the mind supplies you; the mind says it is beautiful. Finished. Now there is no contact with the rose. There is no need; you have said it, now you can move to something else. Without any communion with the rose ... the mind didn't allow you even a glimpse of the rose. The mind came in between, and the heart couldn't come in touch with the rose. Only the heart can say whether it is beautiful or not, because beauty is a feeling, it is not a concept.

You cannot say from the head that it is beautiful. How can you say that? Beauty is not mathematics, it is not measurable. And beauty is not really just in the rose, because to someone else it may not be beautiful at all; and someone else may just pass by without looking at it; and to someone else it may even be ugly. The beauty doesn't exist simply in the rose; the beauty exists in a meeting of the heart with the rose. When the heart meets with the rose, beauty flowers. When the heart comes in deep contact with anything it is a great phenomenon.

If you come in deep contact with any person, the person becomes beautiful. The deeper the contact, the more beauty is revealed. But beauty is a phenomenon that happens to the heart, not to the mind. It is not a calculation, and there is no criterion by which to judge it. It is a feeling.

Heads can argue...

So if I say, 'This rose is not beautiful,' you cannot argue about it. There is no need to argue. You will say, 'That is your feeling. And the rose is beautiful – this is my feeling.' There is no question of argument. Heads can argue. Hearts cannot argue. It is finished, it is a full stop. If I say, 'This is my feeling,' then there is no question of argument.

With the head, argument can continue and we can come to a conclusion. With the heart, the conclusion has already happened. With the heart, there is no procedure towards the conclusion; the conclusion is immediate, instantaneous. With the head, it is a process – you argue, you discuss, you analyse, and then you come to a conclusion about whether this is so or not. With the heart, it is an immediate phenomenon – the conclusion comes first. Look at it: with the head, conclusion comes in the end. With the heart, conclusion comes first, and then you can proceed to find the process – but that is the work of the head.

So when such techniques have to be practised, the first difficulty will be that you don't know what feeling is. Try to develop it. When you touch something, close your eyes; don't think, feel. For example, if I take your hand in my hand and I say to you, 'Close your eyes and feel what is happening,' immediately you will say, 'Your hand is in my hand.' But this is not a feeling, this is a thinking.

Hearts cannot argue...

Then I again say to you, 'Feel. Don't think.' Then you say, 'You are expressing your love.' That too is again thinking. If I insist again, 'Just feel, don't use your head. What are you feeling right now?' only then will you be able to feel and say, `The warmth.' Because love is a conclusion. 'Your hand is in my hand' – this is a head-oriented thought.

The actual feeling is that a certain warmth is flowing from my hand to your hand, or from your hand to my hand. Our life energies are meeting and the point of meeting has become hot, it has become warm. This is the feeling, the sensation, the real. But we go on with the head continuously. That has become a habit; we are trained for it. So you will have to re-open your heart.

Try to live with feelings. Sometimes in the day when you are not doing any particular business – because in business, in the beginning it will be difficult to live with feeling. There, head has proved very efficient, and you cannot depend on feeling. While you are at home playing with your children, the head is not needed, it is not a business – but there too you are with the head. Playing with your children or just sitting with your wife, or not doing anything, relaxing in a chair, feel. Feel the texture of the chair.

Your hand is touching the chair: how are you feeling it? The air is blowing, the breeze is coming in. It touches you. How do you feel? Smells are coming from the kitchen. How do you feel? Just feel. Don't think about them. Don't start brooding that this smell shows that something is being prepared in the kitchen – then you will start dreaming about it. No, just feel whatsoever is the fact. Remain with the fact; don't move in thinking. You are surrounded from everywhere. Everywhere so much is converging on you. The whole existence is coming to meet you from everywhere, from all your senses it is entering you, but

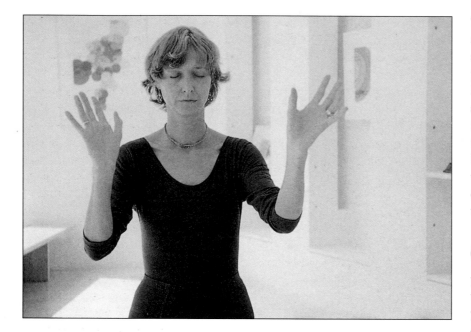

The sound is such, it is so subtle, that you cannot be aware of it unless you focus your awareness towards it. But if you focus your awareness, the whole traffic noise will go far away and the noise of the crow will become the centre. And you will hear it, all the nuances of it – very subtle, but you will be able to hear it.

Grow in sensitivity. When you touch, when you hear, when you eat, when you take a bath, allow your senses to be open. And don't think – feel.

You are standing under the shower: feel the coolness of the water falling on you. Don't think about it. Don't immediately say, `It is very cool. It is cold. It is good.' Don't say anything. Don't verbalise, because the moment you verbalise, you miss feeling. The moment words come in, the mind has started to function. Don't verbalise. Feel the coolness and don't say that it is cool. There is no need to say anything.[9] „

you are in the head, and your senses have become dead; they don't feel.

A certain growth will be needed before you can do this, because this is an inner experiment. If you cannot feel the outer, it will be very difficult for you to feel the inner, because the inner is the subtle. If you cannot feel the gross, you cannot feel the subtle. If you cannot hear the sounds, then it will be difficult for you to hear the inner soundlessness – it will be very difficult. It is so subtle.

You are just sitting in the garden, the traffic is passing by and there are many noises and many sounds. You just close your eyes and try to find the most subtle sound there around you. A crow is cawing: just concentrate yourself on that crow's noise. The whole traffic noise is going on.

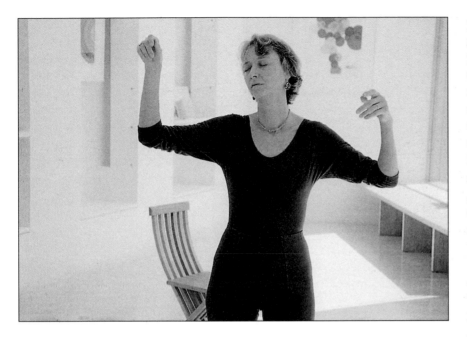

you are making. Your arm goes up into the air, keep your awareness just at the skin where the arm is moving. It suddenly stops – don't pay any attention if the mind tells you to complete the movement, because in fact the movement might want to go in a completely different direction than what the mind has in mind!

It is best to do this without music, so that the music doesn't influence you to follow its rhythm rather than the rhythms of your own body. Try this exercise for just ten or 20 minutes at first, and never do it any longer than 40 minutes. It can be a powerful and liberating release for all kinds of tensions stored in the bodymind – go gently with yourself, and stay alert, following the movement from within.

PICTURED ABOVE AND OPPOSITE:

This exercise is similar to "Latihan," an Indonesian method of allowing the energy of the cosmos to "possess" you. Clear a space so you don't have to worry about bumping into the furniture, stand loose and relaxed, close your eyes or keep them lowered to the ground, not looking at anything in particular. Now just wait, and be inside your body, receptive. After some time you will find that the body wants to move. Allow it – the knack to this exercise is in "allowing" without letting the head come in and interfere. And at the same time remaining aware, so that you don't get so "possessed" that you accidentally hurt yourself. Stay loose, stay in touch with your breathing, and keep your awareness just at the edge of the movements

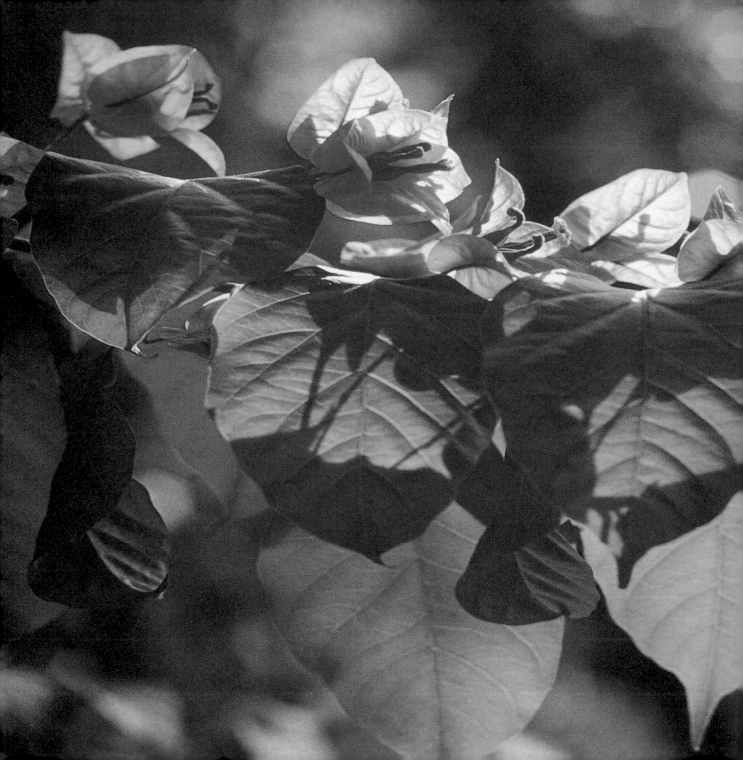

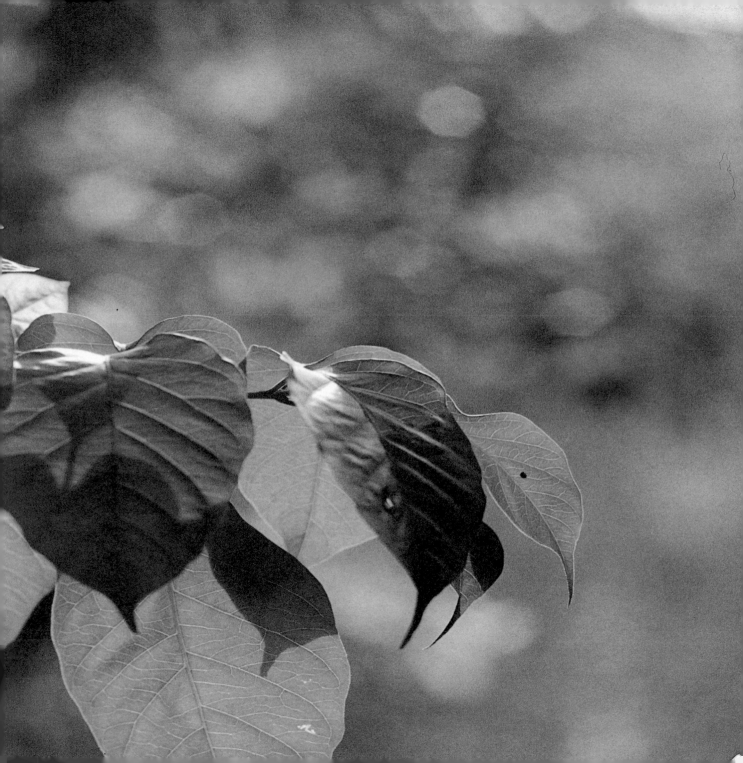

First Things First:
Five Easy Ways to Start Your Day

What's the difference between an optimist and a pessimist? The optimist gets out of bed in the morning, opens the curtains, and says, "Good morning, God!" The pessimist gets out of bed in the morning, opens the curtains, and says, "Good God – morning!"

MORNING.... NO MATTER how you greet it, chances are it is the most routine-bound part of your day. There's something about coming back to the world from a night's journey into sleep that provokes the need for a bit of ritual in even the most unpredictable amongst us. Whether your ritual is simple or complex, whether you hop out of bed like a rabbit or peer out of it like a turtle, depends very much on your temperament. There's no "right" way to be, except the way that feels right for you.

One interesting thing to be aware of, however, is that we all have "sleep cycles" of roughly an hour and a half in duration. That is, we go in and out of deep sleep in a certain rhythm, no matter what our temperament. In a world driven by alarm clocks rather than the natural rhythms of our bodies and the seasons, we can get into a technology-induced difficulty. That is, we can set our alarms to wake us up right in the middle of a deep sleep cycle. Then, no matter what our natural attitude toward morning might be, we will feel groggy, tired, and reluctant to get out of bed.

If you think this might apply to you, try setting your alarm about 45 minutes earlier. The "extra sleep" you're getting right now could be just what's making you feel so tired!

Once you've got your timing sorted out, then try these *Five Easy Ways to Start Your Day*. They're suited to even the most turtle-like slow starters, and are less a shock to the system that starting your day with a cup of black coffee.

Not that we have anything against black coffee, mind you... It's just that it's a good idea to wake yourself up a bit first, so you can be conscious enough to know how much of a good thing to take!

Pull Yourself Up By Your Own Ears

REMEMBER THAT ACUPUNCTURE map in the front of the book, showing the baby curled up in the ear? You can do this while you're still lying in bed, giving that little miniature you in your ear a nice, gentle massage. You can go as fast or as slow as you like, covering all the little curves and crevices, tugging a bit here, tickling a bit there. Massage one ear at a time, or both ears at once. Do it before your mind starts working and distracts you with its list of all the things you've got to do today. Or, if it's too late for that, watch the thoughts passing by while you're doing it – just as if those thoughts belonged to somebody else, or as if you were just listening to them on the radio.

And while we're on the subject of listening, and ears, another nice way to wake up is to take those few moments before you open your eyes to just listen to the sounds. Not just to hear them, but to listen. In a way that Buddhists call *shravan*, 'right listening'. Like this:

> We listen, everyone listens, but right listening is a rare achievement. So what is the difference between listening and right listening, *shravan?*

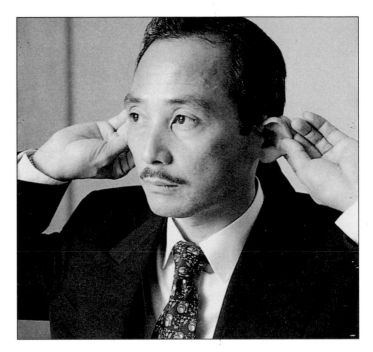

Right listening means not just a fragmentary listening. I am saying something, you are listening to it there. Your ears are being used; you may not be just behind your ears at all; you may have gone somewhere else. You may not be present there. If you are not present there in your totality, then it cannot be right listening. Right listening means you have become just your ears – the whole being is listening. No thinking inside, no thoughts, no thought process, only listening. Try it sometimes; it is a deep meditation in itself. Some birds are singing – the crows – just become listening, forget everything – just be the ears. The wind is passing through the trees, the leaves are rustling; just become the ears, forget everything – no thought process, just listen. Become the ears. Then it is right listening, then your whole being is absorbed into it, then you are totally present.[10]

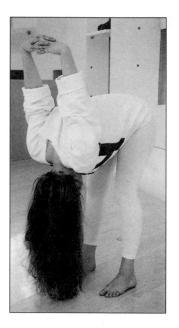

Callisthenics for Lazy People

THIS GROUP OF exercises is specially for those who feel faint at the thought of going to a gym. Or, who tried to follow a work-out video once and kept tripping over their own shoelaces. Or, who would hate to spoil their nice, soft curves by developing unsightly muscle bulges. Not only for those people, mind you – it's just that those people will find these exercises especially attractive. There's no special order to them, and it is absolutely not required that you do them all every morning. You can pick and choose as you like, and design your own lazy callisthenics routine – but do try them all just once, to see for yourself how they feel.

1 This one is great to get the circulation going and clear out the leftover sleep from your head. Stand with your feet comfortably apart, and parallel, with your knees straight. Now, clasp your hands behind your back, palms to the floor and elbows straight. Bend forward from the waist, and let your head hang loose – experiment with seeing how far you can raise your arms up in the back, like the model pictured here. Don't strain or push, and remember to keep breathing. Feel that pleasant stretch down the backs of your arms and legs? Just hang in there with it for a few seconds, and then return – slowly! – to an upright position.

2 This exercise is taken from the Chinese, and is such an effective wake-up call that you might even forget you need that cup of coffee. The movements of the arms are co-ordinated with the breath here – and it works best if you can breathe deep into the belly rather than just into the

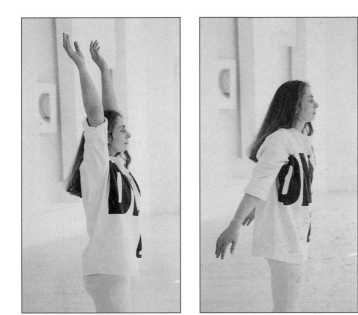

chest, as most of us have learned to do. Inhale through the nose as you raise your arms, keeping your elbows straight and as close to your ears as possible. Exhale through the mouth – pfoooh! – as the arms come back down. The exhalation should quite energetic – pfooooh! – to get rid of as much air as possible before inhaling again through the nose. You can sort of throw your arms down, too, to match the energy of the breath. Repeat a few times, keeping the movment continuous and stop before you get tired or dizzy.

3 Laziness is the key to this one, and letting the movement come from your pelvis. Stand with your feet comfortably apart, and let your arms hang loosely at your sides. You're going to twist from side to side, just

Lazy people have not done any harm in the world. It is the too-active, the hyperactive, who have driven the whole world into misery, madness, slavery. So as far as laziness is concerned, it is very supportive to meditation because meditation needs a very quiet, calm, silent mind. A lazy man is so lazy that he cannot even be bothered to think."

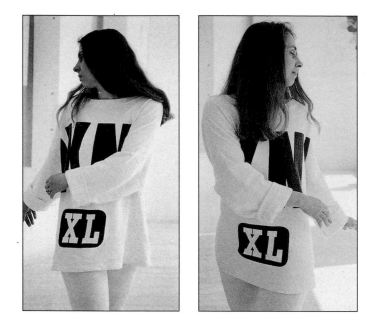

like the common callisthenics exercise – but you're going to be really, really lazy about it! Start the movement at the pelvis, not with the arms. The arms remain loose, and swing naturally as the body moves from side to side. Keep your feet parallel and pointed straight ahead. What we're doing with this exercise is to give the pelvis spine a nice comfortable twist from side to side. Turn your head to follow the movement, as the model is doing in the picture. The tendency will be for the legs to take over the movement – so keep your awareness on initiating the movement from the pelvis, and let everything else follow.

4 The interesting thing about this one is that you get instant feedback whenever you start to space out – you start to topple

Always look at what happens when you do something: if you become peaceful, if you become restful, at home, relaxed, it is right.
This is the criterion, nothing else is criterion.
What is right for you may not be right for somebody else, remember that too.
Because what is easy for you may not be easy for somebody else, something else may be easy for him.
So there can be no universal law about it. Every individual has to work it out for himself.
What is easy for you?[12]

over! A great way to get "centred" before going out to face the cyclone of the day, and to work out the kinks in the knees and the hip joints. Stand with the feet reasonably close together, toes pointed straight ahead. It helps tremendously to focus on a spot on the wall, about eye level, as you raise first one leg and then the other (no, not simultaneously!) and simply swing it forward and backward a few times. There are two versions to this exercise. The one pictured here is to keep your knees straight, and flex them only enough so that your foot doesn't get caught up in the carpet! In another version, where it's actually slightly easier to keep your balance, you can raise your knee as you swing the leg forward and backward.

Experiment with degrees of effort and laziness, point your toes up and then down, etc., whatever feels like a pleasant stretch. If you're like most, you'll notice that every time your mind wanders off

into making plans for the day, wondering what you're going to have for lunch, worrying about that meeting coming up, or whatever, you'll begin to lose your balance. Interesting, mm?

Zen people say that whenever we start thinking of the past or the future, we get "off-centre" – whether it's in our work, our play, our relationships, or in simple physical activities like this one. And any tightrope walker will tell you that the only way they can stay balanced on the rope is by being utterly attentive to where they are in the here and now, and not thinking about where they've been or where they are going. So when you start to topple, bring yourself back to the here and now – and bring your eyes out of that thinking place in your head and back to the spot on the wall. Don't be serious about it, or scold yourself for wandering off. It happens to everybody, and being playful about it is more fun.

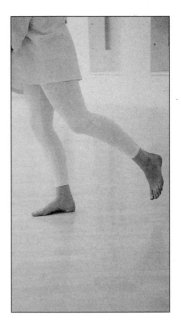

You cannot move away from 'now'. Whatever you do, however fast you run; you will be in the now. And you cannot move in any other space than here. Wherever you will be, that space will become 'here'. We have never moved, as far as our centre is concerned.[13]

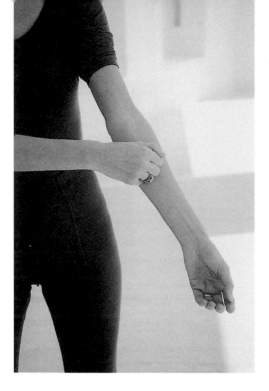

Syncopated Rhythms

THIS WORKS BEST if you actually follow a set progression as we have pictured here – just to help you make sure you don't leave any part of you out. What you're doing is waking up all the energy meridians in the body. How you're doing it is easily and gently, with a light-hearted attitude as if you're playing 'pat-a-cake.' You'll be gathering your hands into loose fists, and giving all the meridian lines a soft pounding. Start with the back of the neck and shoulders, remembering to keep your shoulders loose – are you breathing? – and using both fists. Next, go to one arm (right or left, your choice!) and, using the opposite fist, work your way thoroughly from top to bottom on the inside of the arm, and then up on the outside, three times in

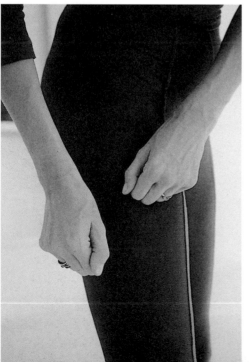

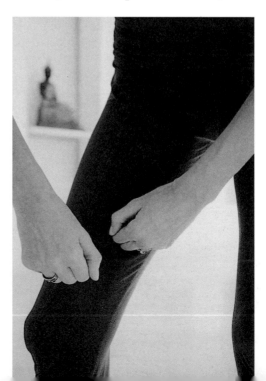

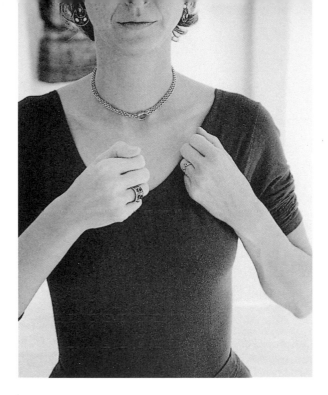

A gentle pounding of the energy meridians is a pleasant and refreshing wake-up for the body after a night's sleep. While doing the exercise, be sure to follow the direction of the movement of energy through the meridians, as indicated in the instructions below.

all. When you've finished with one arm, move across your chest, using both fists and remembering to be gentle. Work your way across to the other arm, which you pound as before, a total of three times. Now revisit your chest again briefly and move down the front of the torso. Down the front of the pelvic area, and over to one leg – are you a bit ticklish where your leg meets your body? Down the outside of the leg and up the inside, using both fists and again making the circle three times. Finish up with the buttocks and the kidney area, a gentle sort of circular pounding for as long as it takes to create a sense of warmth and relaxation within yourself. Shake out your hands to finish.

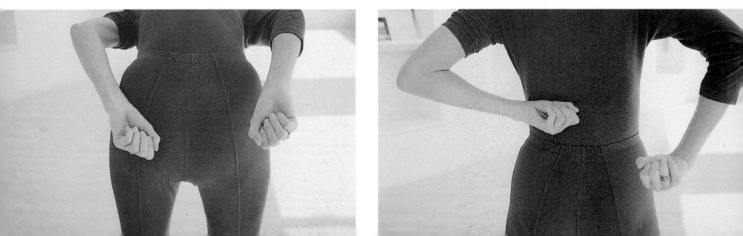

Yoga Wake-Ups for Weekday Warriors

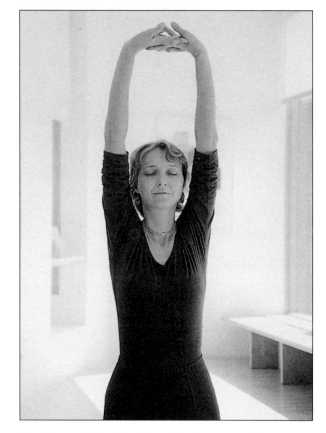

MAYBE YOU THINK the preceding exercises are too easy. Maybe you're of the "no pain, no gain" school and can't imagine that just playing around like that will do you any good. Or, maybe you like the preceding exercises, but want to add something a little more strenuous to your routine.

If you do them properly, the two exercises pictured on these pages shouldn't cause you any pain – sorry, folks – but they will require you to reach just a little higher, try just a little harder, stretch just a little more. They are designed for the "do-ers" among us, the ones who always climbed to the highest branches of the trees when they were children. That doesn't mean the lazy ones among us can't try them, too. They aren't that difficult, after all....

A special note for weekday warriors, here and everywhere – when you're doing any exercise that involves stretching, please do stop short of actually causing yourself pain. There's a point where it "hurts good," where the stretch is pleasurably painful, but not just painfully painful. Find that place, stay in it as long as you like, but don't go beyond it. Okay?

1 If you've tried the previous breathing exercise, you'll notice right away that this one gives you a different kind of feeling. Raise your arms above your head and clasp your hands with the palms turned upward. Keeping the arms raised, and checking to see that the shoulders are relaxed, inhale and exhale, deeply and slowly, through the nose. Keep your elbows as close together as possible, and your spine straight. The exercise can bring a lot of energy to the head, so if it begins to cause dizziness, stop and sit down.

2/3 Have you seen how a dog stretches when he gets up after a nap? This exercise is designed to duplicate that luxurious, spine-opening

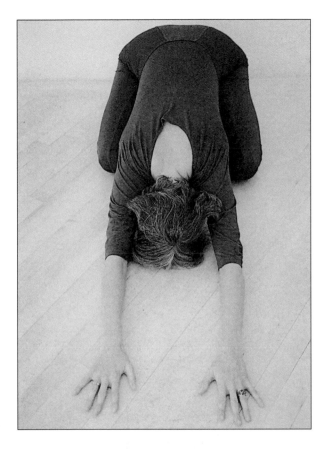

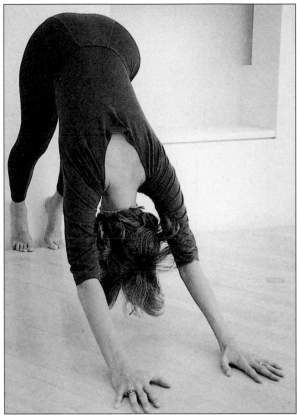

stretch of the dog. Clear enough space so that you can lie face down with your arms outstretched and your feet against a wall. Easily and gently, however it works best for you, raise your body up so the buttocks form the bottom of an upside-down V-shape as shown by our model in the first photo. Let your weight really rest on your arms, and don't make your spine and neck do the work. Rather, keep your spine straight but let your body "hang loose" being supported by the arms, and relaxing and opening more and more. Slowly slowly, feeling the stretching and taking it as far as it feels comfortable but no more, move your feet so they are flat on the floor, heels against the wall. Feel that stretch at the back of your legs? Let yourself down easy, and repeat as many times as you like. Note: People with back problems should check with their doctors before trying this.

The Great Shower Escape

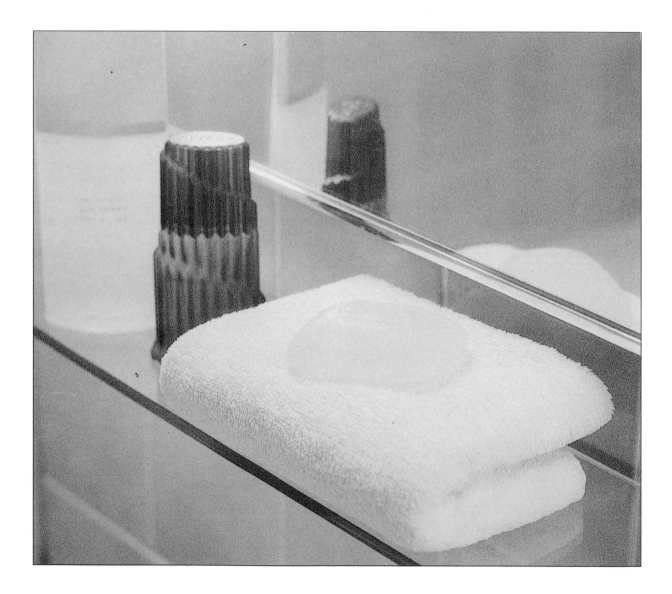

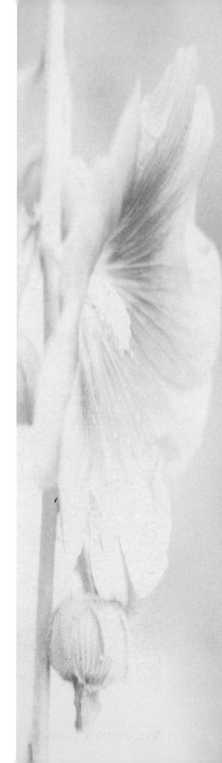

From this moment, start loving yourself, be more tender to yourself. Don't be hard, don't be cruel! Give a little joy to your body, to your mind. It is your mind and you have to take care of it. It is your body; treat it as a temple. And small things make much difference....

You take a shower every day: you can do it very unconcernedly, you can do it very lovingly. You can feel the water falling on the body. You can enjoy the feel, the freshness, the joy that comes to the body — how every cell of the body starts feeling fresh. You can enjoy — it is your body: your body is feeling good.

Love, eat, work and enjoy! Enjoy small moments. Small things are there: sipping tea or coffee or just lying on the bed and relaxing, enjoy! And make them so tremendously enjoyable that they become almost divine, sacred.[14]

COMMUTER WORKOUTS
Making the Most of To-ing and Fro-ing

THE NEXT TIME you're on you way to work in the morning, step back a little and have a look around at your fellow commuters. Frightening, isn't it? It's just like a low-budget science fiction movie, one of those where human bodies are being occupied by Zombies from Galaxy B29X47. Pretty soon a strange, metallic voice is going to take over all the radio and television stations and instruct everybody to start manufacturing Brussels sprouts, or whatever it is they so desperately need back there.

Why do we all look so... soulless when we're on our way to work? Is it because we're not properly awake yet? Is it because we are so much in dread of the day ahead of us? It might be a little of both those things, but most of all it's because commuting to and from work tends to be one of the most unproductive, burdensome things we do. It's a kind of neither-this-nor-that time, where we are neither free to play and enjoy ourselves, nor are we able to get any work done. So we put ourselves in a kind of suspended animation and wait for the thing to be over.

This section of *BodyWisdom* explores some ways you can start to use that "dead time" of commuting to help yourself feel more alive. We've tried to cover every possible commuting situation – from walking, to taking the bus or the train, to driving. About the only thing we haven't covered is riding a bicycle, a scooter or motorbike – we figure you need your total attention in that form of transport so you don't get yourself killed! But every other alternative gives you so many opportunities to relax, take it easy, and arrive at your destination looking like a human being instead of a Zombie from Galaxy B29X47.

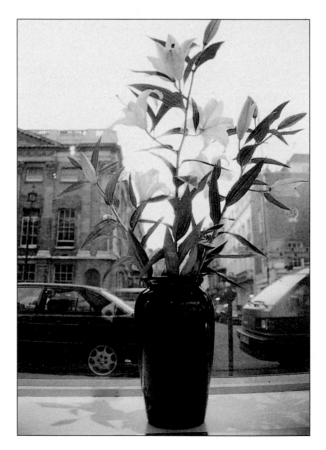

It's All In How You Look At It

REMEMBER THE FIRST time you ever went alone on a really big journey? It might have been when your parents finally allowed you to go down to the corner by yourself on your bicycle, or the first time you flew alone on a plane, it doesn't matter. What's important to remember is that feeling of excitement and adventure, that freshness in your eyes, that sense that you could be anybody you wanted to be, because nobody knew who you were or had any ideas about you.

Now, we're not seriously suggesting that you can recover that lost innocence every single time you step out your door to go to work, are we?

Well, why not? At least you could give it a try, there's nothing to lose after all and a whole landscape of wonder to gain. If you walk to the bus stop or to the train station, do you pass any gardens on the way? Take notice of what's coming into bloom, what's fading and falling to the ground, how the leaves are changing colour or how they reflect the morning sun. Today is not just like every other day, or we'd all be in trouble. The Zombies from Galaxy B29X47 would have already taken over. No gardens, you say? You live in the middle of the city and there's no plant life to be found? Then look at the faces of people on the street – how diverse, how many moods and feelings they have... see if you can imagine what their kitchen looks like, whether they have children or pet goldfish. Make up stories about them in your head.

If it seems too risky to look at their faces (it can seem like that, these days, we realise) then look at their shoes – what does the person look like who wears those shoes? – and take a quick look to see if you've come anywhere close. Give yourself points every time you see something purple, make a fool of yourself and kick a rock down the sidewalk for a whole block.

Set up a different experiment for yourself every day for a week. One day just turn your whole attention to the sounds of the street, with all their textures and harmonies and dissonance. The second day, take notice of the smells and fragrances, of shrubbery and soil, of cafes and the traffic. Take each of your senses and give them their own day to play, and show to you what they can do.

There are hundreds of opportunities to marvel at life between where you live and where you work. Just because you haven't taken any notice of them doesn't mean they aren't there.

The point is, there's life all around and we're missing 90 percent of it when we get so busy in our heads making a mental list for the 15th time, thinking about what we said to so-and-so and what we should have said, etc. on and on... you know the story. Give yourself a break. Pretend you're in Paris, or in another century, or setting out on a journey to Galaxy B29X47 to take over the bodies of all the Zombies and make them dance. Create your own adventure, the world is never as dull as it seems. It's all in how you look at it.

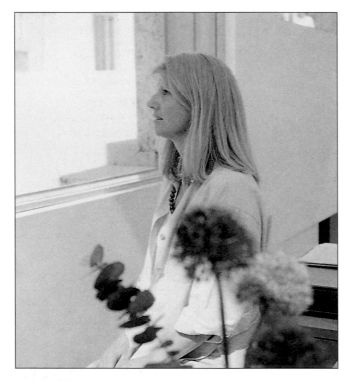

Step by Step by Step

MEDITATION IS REALLY just being able to watch, to make contact with, observe, and respond from that space within ourselves that hasn't changed since the days when we were children, and won't change as we grow older. It's a space that different cultures and religions have given different names to — the soul, the Self with a capital S, the *atman*, to name a few. It's who we are when we aren't any of the labels we put on ourselves — or any of the labels put on us by others. It's where our BodyWisdom lives, and our capacity for unconditional love. It's where we journey to when we are most deeply asleep, and it's where people live when they have become so absolutely awake that they have neither dreams nor any need for them.

The journey into meditation is easiest when it starts simply, by learning to watch what is closest to us. And, one of the closest things to us which we can observe is our own body and its movements. Getting to work and back home again is something we all get the knack of pretty quickly, once we've done it a few times. That's why we can put the whole journey on automatic pilot and think about other things.

As you walk, just walk. Feel your feet. Feel how first the heel, then the middle of the foot, then the ball of the foot touches the ground. Go slowly, and then more quickly. See if you can stay with the awareness of your feet touching the ground.

Tell yourself that you will stop – Stop! – when you hear the sound of a horn, or the barking of a dog. Do it, no matter how silly it looks, and just be there, in that Stop! for a few seconds before you carry on.

Go to your car and open the door as if you are opening it for the first time, as if you are not really sure how the door handle works. Pull the door open slowly, listening to the sound it makes. Notice all the different smells inside the car, the upholstery, the plastics and the metal.

Watch how you get into the car – as much as possible not changing your movements from those you normally make. Put the key in the ignition, feeling all the little nuances of how it fits. Start the car, noticing what you do with the gas pedal.

At every step, see if you can watch the movements your body normally makes automatically, reaching for the gear shift or the seat belt, turning to look behind you, hunching your shoulders, revving the engine, adjusting the mirror... what does that automatic pilot normally do when you aren't paying any attention? How many little unnecessary movements, what kinds of unconscious routines, sensible and insensible are you making?

As you stand waiting for the bus, see if you can just stand there watching your breath, not being impatient, not looking up the street to see if the bus is coming. Just the breath, in and out, in and out. Whenever your mind wanders off, or you find yourself wanting to look at your watch, acknowledge the impulse, take care of it, and then go back to watching your breath.

There are so many opportunities to watch, to meditate. No need to chant mantras, or sit in the lotus position. Whenever you are watching, alert, aware of what you're doing, you're in meditation.

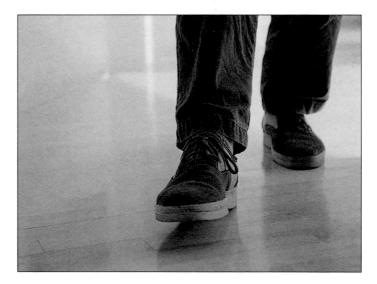

Space Among the Sardines

AS WE BECOME more sensitive, we become more and more aware of how much we are all affected by one another. We all have the experience of it, really, even though we might not have ever given it much thought. Maybe we have a friend who we just love being around because they have such a light-hearted approach to life, or somebody at work we avoid because they are always in a complaining mood. Some people have the knack of putting others at ease, while others seem to spark conflict and tension wherever they go.

This capacity to affect each other is not just in the words we speak or the actions we take — it happens on many levels. When we say somebody "has a weird vibe" we're not necessarily referring to what they say or do. More often, we're talking about something non-verbal, a little bit hidden and mysterious. Somehow we are feeling the effect of this person's thoughts and feelings, and our discomfort might even come from the sense that what's going on beneath the surface of the person is at odds with their outward behavior. In other words, it's not just physical diseases that are contagious, it's thoughts and feelings, too.

Different people have different needs for what's sometimes called "personal space." You've probably experienced this, when talking to somebody at a party for example. The person seems to be right in your face, and if you don't actually, physically back away from them you keep having the feeling you'd like to. The amount of distance between people that feels comfortable in social interaction tends to vary with different cultures, too. If you stand in a crowded elevator in China, for example, you'll experience a completely different "vibe" than you will under the same conditions in Chicago. In China people are more self-contained, more at ease in shoulder-to-shoulder situations. The silence that is strained and tense in the Chicago elevator becomes noticeably more relaxed and at ease in China.

So we get to the point of the story, which is that if you commute to work in a moving can of sardines, it will help you cope if you can become Chinese. We can create a lot of tension in the body by trying to shrink away from our fellow-passengers. If you can experiment with being Chinese, your need for personal, physical space will shrink. Try it — as soon as you manage to squeeze yourself in place, consciously relax your body, starting with the shoulders and letting yourself settle into your feet (or into your seat) just as you might as if there were nobody else around. Close your eyes, or keep them slightly unfocused and turned downwards. Now imagine that you are expanding into the space just surrounding your body, just flowing into it with every outbreath, taking more space for yourself. That person's elbow in your back doesn't have to be an elbow, it could be the knot of an old tree. All it is, really, when you take your mind out of it, is a sensation of pressure, maybe of warmth. Relax, it's a great opportunity to just be at home in yourself with nothing in particular to do. And you might just find that your relaxation spreads to your fellow passengers — it's contagious!

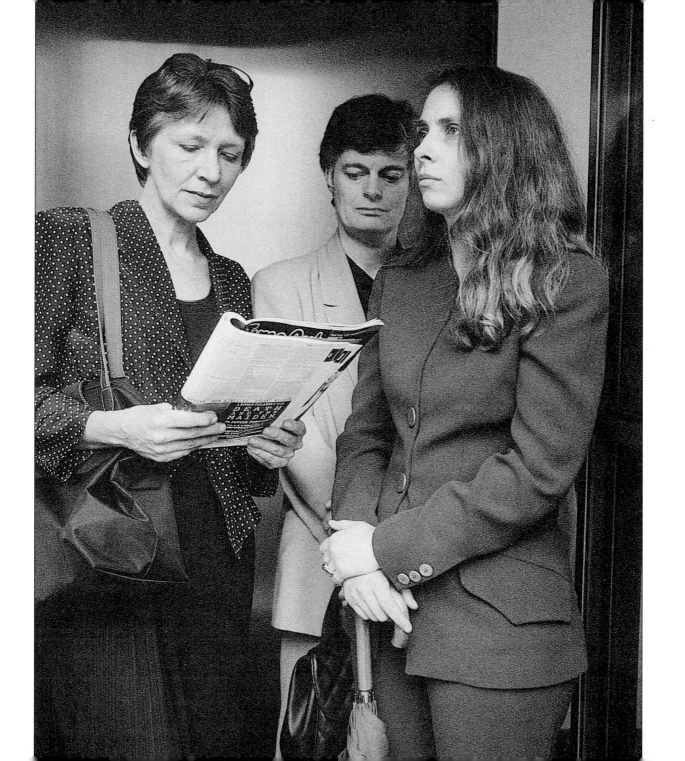

Just Standing Around

AGAIN AND AGAIN we will be coming back to the point that there are a thousand and one everyday opportunities to relax, to make contact with the body and feel how it is doing and what it needs, to bring a quality of meditation and alertness to what you are doing. Why? Because tension and stress is aggravated by not being in contact with our bodies and our feelings, by getting so caught up in the rat race that we lose track of our own rhythms.

The following exercises come from Osho's talks with people who came to see him about their own problems and tensions and difficulties. They are just small things you can do whenever you think about them throughout the day. But we put them here in the "Commuter Workouts" section because moving from one place to another is a good opportunity to remember to do them. The first will help in getting your feet on the ground. You could do it standing on the train platform, or waiting for a bus... even in that crowded elevator, if you like!

1 Stand on your feet, just six or eight inches apart, and close your eyes. Then put your whole weight first on the right foot, as if you are standing only on the right. The left is unburdened. Feel it... and then shift to the left foot. Have the whole burden on the left and relieve the right completely, as if it has nothing to do. It is just there on the earth but it has no weight on it.

Do this four or five times – feeling this shift of energy – and feel how it feels. Then try to be just in the middle, neither on the left or the right, or on both. Just in the middle, no emphasis, fifty-fifty. That 50/50 feeling will give you more rootedness in the earth.[15]

2 This one adds a little more depth to the previous exercise of walking consciously, taking it a little bit farther to encompass more movements and activities that we usually do without being aware of them. There's a bit of extra encouragement in it, too ... and a description of the more subtle benefits to be gained from doing these simple exercises.

As you grow in consciousness the world itself starts changing. Nothing needs to be done directly; all the changes that happen are almost of their own accord. Only one thing that is needed is an effort to be more conscious. Start becoming more and more conscious of everything that you are doing. Walking, walk consciously; bring your total attention to walking. And there is a great difference between when you just walk without any consciousness and when you bring the quality of consciousness to walking. The change is radical. It may not be visible from the outside, but from the inside it is really moving into another dimension.
Try some small act: for example, moving your hand. You can move it mechanically – then move it with great consciousness, feeling the movement, slowly,

slowly, looking from the inside at how you are moving it. In this small gesture you are on the threshold of god, because a miracle is happening. It is one of the greatest mysteries which science has not yet been able to fathom.

You decide that you should move the hand and the hand follows your decision. It is a miracle because it is consciousness contacting matter, and not only that, but matter following consciousness. The bridge has not yet been found – it is magic! It is the power of the mind over matter; that's what magic is all about. You do it the whole day, but you have not done it consciously; otherwise in this simple gesture a great meditation will arise in you. This is the way god is moving the whole existence; in this small gesture is the whole history of existence.

The scriptures say that god said, "Let there be light" and there was light. Now, it looks utter nonsense if you think about it logically. How can there be light just by saying "Let there be light"? But this is happening every day continuously! When you say "Let there be a movement in my hand" and the hand moves, it is the same miracle.[16]

3 When we talked about finding "Space Among the Sardines" did you have trouble imagining that you could ever relax while crammed into a tunnel with hundreds of other commuters? Does the very "vibe" of rush hour make you feel exhausted, no matter what you do? It might be that you are really particularly susceptible to the tensions and energies of other people, and need a little extra help to protect yourself. Here's what Osho suggested to one person who said she always became exhausted when

she had to be around lots of people engaged in the sort of busyness that surrounds most of us every working day.

Every night before you go to sleep, just sit in the bed and imagine an aura around your body, just six inches away from your body, the same shape as the body, surrounding you, protecting you. It will become a shield. Just do it for four, five minutes, and then, still feeling it, go to sleep. Fall into sleep imagining that aura like a blanket around you which protects you so that no tension can enter from the outside, no thought can enter from the outside; no outside vibrations can enter you. Just feeling that aura, fall asleep.

This has to be done the last thing at night. After it, simply go to sleep so the feeling continues in your unconscious. That is the whole thing – the whole mechanism is that you start by consciously imagining, then you start falling asleep. By and by when you are on the threshold of sleep, a little imagination continues, lingers on. You fall asleep but that little imagination enters the unconscious. That becomes a tremendous force and energy.

I don't see that the problem is within you. The problem is coming from the outside. You don't have a protective aura. It happens to many people, because we don't know how to protect ourselves from others. Others are not only there – they are broadcasting their being continuously in subtle vibrations. If a tense person passes by you, he is simply throwing arrows of tension all around – not particularly addressed to you; he is simply throwing. And he is unconscious; he is not doing it to anybody knowingly. He has to throw it because he is too burdened. He will go mad if he doesn't throw it. It is not that he has decided to throw it, it is overflowing. It is too much and he cannot contain it, so it goes on overflowing.

Somebody passes by you and he goes on throwing something at you. If you are receptive and you don't have a protective aura.... And meditation makes one receptive, very receptive. So when you are alone, it is good; when you are surrounded by meditative people, very good. But when you are in the world, in the marketplace, and people are not meditative but are very tense, anxious, have a thousand and one strains on their mind, then you just start getting them. And you are vulnerable; meditation makes one very soft, so whatsoever comes, enters.

After meditation one has to create a protective aura. Sometimes it happens automatically, sometimes it doesn't. It is not happening automatically to you, so you have to work for it. It will be coming within three months. Any time between three weeks and three months, you will start feeling very, very powerful. So in the night, fall asleep thinking this way. In the morning the first thought has to be again this. The moment you become aware that now sleep is gone, don't open your eyes. Just feel your aura all over the body protecting you. Do it for four, five minutes again, and then get up. When you are taking your bath and your tea, go on remembering it. Then in the daytime also whenever you feel you

have time – sitting in a car or a train, or in the office doing nothing – just again relax into it. For a single moment feel it again.

Between three weeks and three months you will start feeling it almost like a solid thing. It will surround you and you will be able to feel that you can now pass through a crowd and you will remain unaffected, untouched. It will make you tremendously happy because now only your problems will be your problems, nobody else's.

It is very easy to solve one's own problems because they are one's own. It is very difficult when you go on getting others' problems; then you cannot solve them, because in the first place they don't belong to you. Many people come to me and they say they had some problem but suddenly here it is gone. It was never their problem – otherwise it cannot go. It must have been somebody else's. They must have been stepfathering it, fostering it. It must have entered from somebody else's mind. But people are so unaware that they don't know what is theirs and what is the others. Everything goes on getting into a mess.

You don't have many problems, and you will be able to solve your problems; that is not a big thing. This time try to create a protective aura – and you will be able to see it and its function. You will see that you are completely protected. Wherever you go, things will be coming to you but they will be returned; they will not touch you.[17]

Fly, Fly High

THE FOLLOWING MEDITATION WAS GIVEN BY OSHO TO AN AIRLINE PILOT. BUT IT'S GREAT FOR ANYBODY WHO FLIES A LOT IN THE COURSE OF THEIR WORK... ADAPT THE DETAILS TO MAKE SENSE TO YOUR OWN SITUATION, AND ENJOY THE RIDE!

YOU CANNOT FIND a better situation to meditate than while flying.... The higher the altitude, the easier is the meditation; hence, for centuries, meditators have been moving to the Himalayas to find a high altitude.

When the gravitation is less and the earth is very far away, many of the downward pulls of the earth are far away. You are far away from the corrupted society that man has built. You are surrounded by clouds and the stars and the moon and the sun and the vast space.... So do one thing: start feeling one with that vastness, and do it in three steps.

The first step is: for a few minutes just think that you are becoming bigger... you are filling the whole cabin of the plane.

Then the second step: start feeling that you are becoming even bigger, bigger than the plane, in fact the plane is now inside you — the second step.

And the third step: feel that you have expanded into the whole sky. Now these clouds that are moving by outside the window, and the moon, and the stars – they are moving in you: you are huge, unlimited. This feeling will become your meditation, and you will feel completely relaxed and non-tense.... You will get down from the flight more fresh than you had begun. And keep quiet – don't talk with people unless it is necessary....

In fact in the early days – when the airplane was just invented – the thrill of the airplane was the thrill of the sky. But we go on losing things because they become too routine. Now you are flying every day, so who looks at the sky and who looks at the sun making beautiful psychedelic colours on the clouds – who looks?

So start looking at the sky that surrounds you there and by and by let there be a meeting between the inner sky and the outer sky...

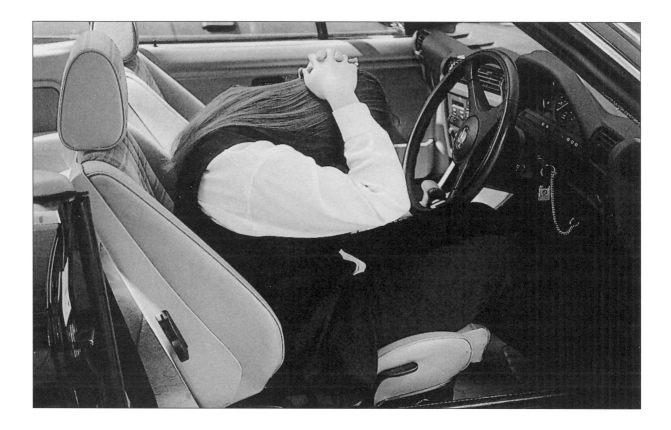

Helpful Hints for Taking to the Road

THERE ARE A lot more opportunities to experiment with different kinds of meditations when you're being taken somewhere, than when you have to be in the driver's seat. But when it's your own car, at least you have the right to make some adjustments in the environment so that your journey is as pleasant as possible. You can choose the radio station, or listen to your favorite music or a talking book. If you weren't concerned about whether people would see you, you could even sing along with your favourite songs, talk to yourself, tell yourself stories. Come to think of it, why are you concerned about whether people will see you? The worst that can happen is that they'll think you have a few screws loose (probably just envious of your carefree spontaneity, really) and no matter what they think, chances are they'll never see you again.

The other thing that's in your control when you're driving is what you do with your body. Believe it or not, those hunched-up shoulders and that tension running all the way from your hip down to your foot on the accelerator will not help you to respond more quickly to an emergency. Just the opposite, in fact – when our bodies are locked in tension it takes them longer to react. So as you're barrelling down the motorway remind yourself frequently to check the shoulders and legs to see that they're relaxed and loose. If they're all tensed up, take a deep breath and let the tension go with the outbreath. Check your hands on the steering wheel, too – are you clutching onto it as though you were saving yourself from a 100 foot drop down onto the rocks below? Let go a little bit, there are no rocks, there is no below.

Many, many people who do a lot of driving develop lower back problems. If you can manage to keep yourself more relaxed it will help – and the newer cars are getting more body-friendly all the time. But even the best-designed seat is made for the "average" person, and most of us aren't average. Even if your back is fine, experiment with using a pillow for support, trying out different sizes and firmness till you find one that makes you say "A-a-a-ah" when you get behind the wheel, and still feels good when you arrive.

Finally, try out the exercise pictured opposite. Do it first thing, when you get into the car, when you're stuck in an unmoving traffic jam, and when you reach your destination. Just clasp your hands and put them on the back of your head, as shown. Let the weight of your hands pull your head forward, feeling the stretching that happens in your neck and all the way down your spine. Don't pull down, just relax your arms and let the weight of your hands do all the work. "A-a-a-ah."

" A WISE MAN lives moment to moment, he has no planning. His life is just free like a cloud floating in the sky, not going to some goal, not determined. He has no map for the future, he lives without a map, he moves without a map; because the real thing is not the goal, the real thing is the beauty of the movement. The real thing is not reaching, the real thing is the journey. Remember, the real thing is the journey, the very travelling. It is so beautiful, why bother about the goal? The journey is life and it is an infinite journey. You have been on the move from the very beginning – if there was any beginning. Those who know say there was no beginning, so from no beginning you have been on the move, to the no end you will be on the move – and if you are goal-oriented, you will miss. The whole is the journey, the path, the endless path, never beginning, never ending. There is really no goal – goal is created by the cunning mind. Where is this whole existence moving? Where? It is not going anywhere. It is simply going, and the go-ing is so beautiful, that is why existence is unbur-dened. There is no plan, no goal, no purpose. It is not a business, it is a play, a *leela*. Every moment is the goal.[18] "

Office Routines: Quick Breaks from Life in the Fast Lane

EVEN A CASUAL glance into the average office is enough to make it painfully obvious why so many people today are suffering from stress-related aches and pains. Everybody has a mountain of papers piled on their desks, over which they are crouched like trolls. This one is clutching the phone in one hand, a calendar in the other, and searching frantically in her drawer for a pencil, and that one looks like he's been staring into the computer screen for so long he's got bytes for brains. The guy in the corner pouring himself a cup of coffee seems to have misplaced his neck somewhere in the depths of his shoulders, and the woman sitting at the desk with the highest mountain looks like she carries the whole thing home on her shoulders every night, only to bring it back to the same place every morning.

But, as burdensome as this picture is, it seems unlikely that we're going to be able to do very much, very soon, about changing the amount of work we have, or the time available for us to do it. Who on earth has time for the exercise we are told our bodies need to be more relaxed and healthy? Some people use the lunch hour to go to the health club, or manage to squeeze in a run or a workout at the beginning or the end of the day. But there are many things we can do throughout the day that will not just help our bodies feel better, but will actually help us accomplish more in the available time, in a more relaxed and enjoyable way.

This section is full of things you can do to take a quick break from your "life in the fast lane." Things to retrieve your neck from the depths of your shoulders, to clear your head for that important meeting coming up, to retrieve your mind from the innards of the computer and to wake yourself up without having to drink another cup of that lethal coffee. Start with the exercise represented on the opposite page, right now – it's the quickest break of all, and once you get the knack it's amazingly refreshing. It goes like this:

Imagine there is a clear plastic hose filled with running water that goes from the bottom of your spine (where it meets your chair as you sit) to the top of your head. Once you've got the hose in your imagination, check it out: does it have any kinks in it anywhere that are keeping the water from flowing freely? If so, just make whatever small, subtle adjustments are needed in how you're sitting, to unkink the hose so the water can flow.

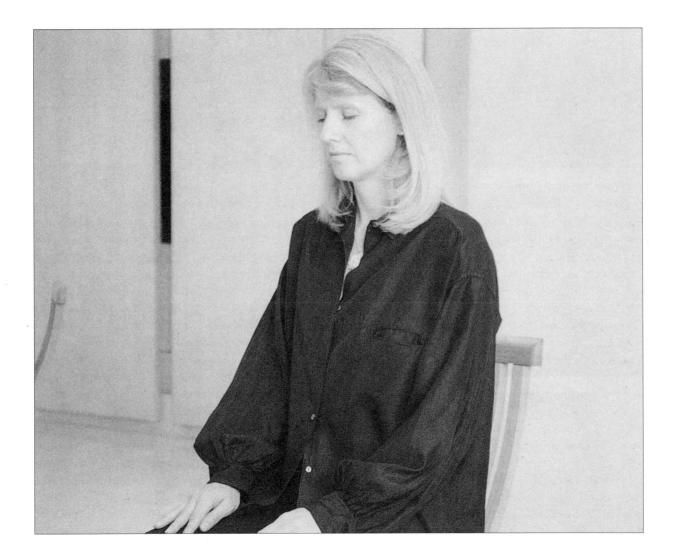

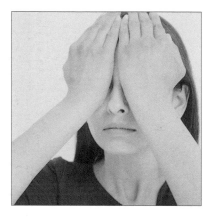

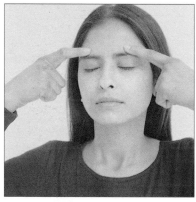

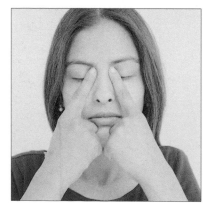

When the Eyes Have Had It

THE EYES GIVE us perhaps the most obvious and visible example of the body's natural wisdom. They keep themselves clean and moist by blinking, they produce tears to wash out harmful intruders, and they expand and contract so we can see in different kinds of light and at different distances – all without any need of conscious direction from the mind. They are smart in other ways too: if you watch people, and take note of what you do yourself, you can see that the eyes have an extraordinary talent for persuading us to do exactly the right thing to help them refresh and renew themselves when they are tired.

Most of the pictures on these pages will look familiar to anybody who has taken note of what we do when our eyes are tired. What you might not know, however, is that all these little unconscious moves have a specific healing purpose within the ancient healing system of shiatsu. So if you start applying these techniques consciously, with more awareness of how they can help you, they will naturally be even more effective.

1 Cup your hands over your eyes, gently but firmly so your eyes are free to open but no light gets in. Do you see all those fireworks and streaks of light? That means your eyes have been working overtime.

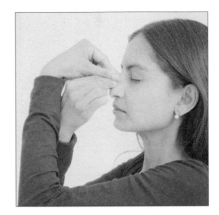

2 These points are located the width of one finger above the middle of the eyebrow, in line with the pupils as you look straight ahead. No need to dig your thumbs in – just a light pressure will do, for about half a minute. This is also very good to do when you feel a bit fuzzy-headed and tense around the face and neck.

3 Use very gentle pressure here, in the little hollows that just fit your fingers, right above the tear ducts. Keep the pressure steady for about thirty seconds, don't forget to breathe, and check to see that your shoulders are relaxed.

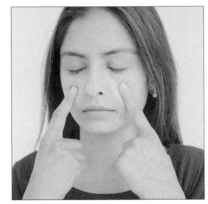

4 You've seen people do this one when they take off their glasses after a gruelling session with the Sunday papers, right? Start at the top, and pull all that tension from between your eyebrows right down and off the tip of your nose.

5 This one is called "Facial Beauty" in shiatsu, and is also good for stuffy noses, headaches, toothaches and sinus troubles. Press upwards on the cheekbones from below, at the point just under the pupils of the eyes, and hold for about half a minute.

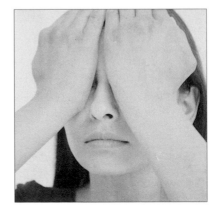

6 Now cup your hands over your eyes again, as you did at the beginning. Notice how much darker and more peaceful it is in there now? That's the language your eyes use when they want to say thank you.

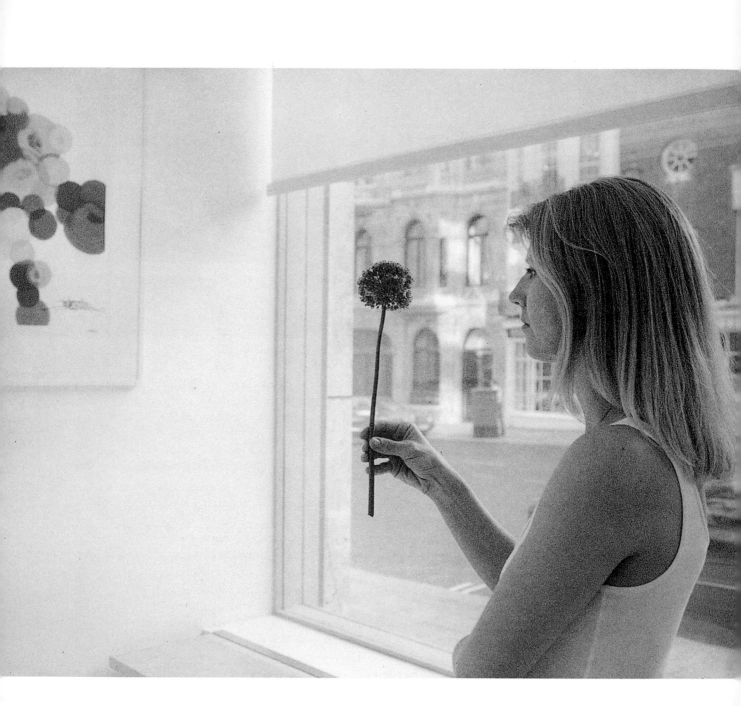

Taking a Different Perspective

IF YOU'RE APPROACHING middle age and have noticed that your arms are getting too short to allow you to read the newspaper properly, don't be surprised. Our eyes can lose flexibility as we get older, just like our bodies can. And it probably happens to more people these days than it used to, because when we sit at a desk most of the time, our eyes don't get very many opportunities to flex their muscles. In fact, it's become such a common phenomenon, and happens in such a predictable way, that eye charts have been developed that can tell you with remarkable accuracy just how old you are, depending on how far away you have to hold the chart to read it.

About 25 years ago, a man named Gregory Bates decided that he, for one, wasn't going to just resign himself to the poor eyesight that afflicts so many people, whether it comes from ageing or from other factors such as habitual tension in the eyes. He developed a series of exercises and published them in a book called *Sight Without Glasses* and hundreds of thousands of people have benefitted from his work. We've pictured just one of his methods here, which will help you give your eyes a little stretch from time to time as you make your way through the day.

The idea is to shift your focus from a near object to one that is far away, and then back again. Back and forth, just a few times, until you can see both points clearly and without feeling a strain. Our model here is doing this exercise with a flower and a painting – but it is even more effective if you have two objects that are quite similar. A clock on your desk, and a clock on the wall, for example, or a calendar, will let you explore the flexibility of your vision in a more systematic way. Can you see the numbers equally well, both close up and far away?

Another variation to add to this experiment, which does not come from Bates but rather from a suggestion made by Osho, is to see what happens when you stop looking through your eyes, and start looking from behind them. Don't think too much about what that means, or the mechanics of it, just give it a try. Look from behind your eyes, not through them. Feel the difference, and see if it makes any difference in how well you can see.

Airing Out the Headroom

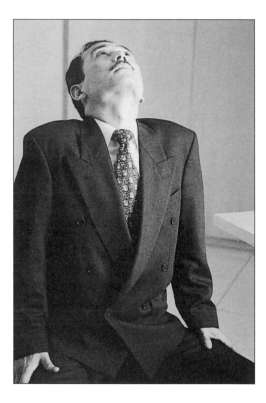

JUST A COUPLE of generations ago, most people worked with their hands and their bodies. Nowadays, most of us work with just our heads. It can get pretty crowded in there, with 15 projects going on at once, two or three people having a heated debate, and a couple of folks running around trying to retrieve something they have the feeling they've lost, but they're not sure what it is. If we don't give our heads a break from time to time, all that busyness can start overflowing and causing trouble in the neck and shoulders, and from there down

to the back, or into the belly – all kinds of places where it doesn't belong. And then we're much more tired at the end of our seven-hour day than grandad ever was doing his 12-hour day on the farm.

The exercises in this section are all designed to give the brain a break, to chase everybody out for just a few seconds so the cleaning lady can come in. To call a

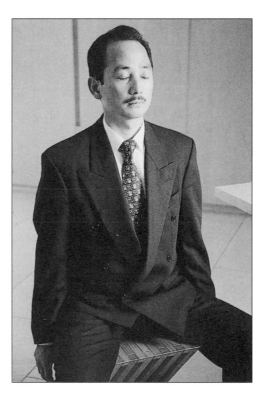

time-out and give everybody a chance to go splash a little water on their faces and get ready for the next round.

Start as pictured here, by giving your shoulders a really exaggerated shrug, as if not only don't you know, you really *really* don't know, you are absolutely *clueless*. What you're doing here is exaggerating the tension that exists already, taking it to the max, really scrunching yourself up like a used piece of paper ready to toss in the bin. Then tilt your head right back, as far as it will go. As you do it, you might notice that one side of your neck somehow feels more bulky than the other, which means it's holding more tension – most probably on the side of your preferred hand. Inhale as you scrunch up, and then exhale as you let it go. Let it go just like that – plop! – all of a sudden let go. That sense of heat in the back of the neck and shoulders is your blood flowing through there again – congratulations!

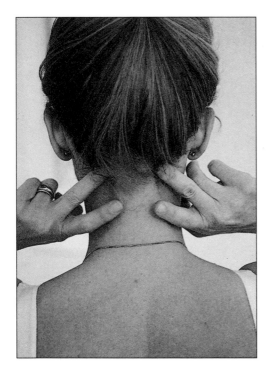

The "gates of consciousness" can be found by searching for small hollows just beneath the bony ridge of the skull.

THESE TWO PICTURES are to help you find the shiatsu points that will help you think a little clearer, be a little more alert, a little less confused. The points shown in the picture on the left are called "gates of consciousness" and are located just on the underside of that bony ridge there in the back. As you tilt your head back a little, you can feel the hollows there. Explore around with your fingers until you find the right place – it's a little different on everybody but you'll know where it is because when you find it your fingers will nestle in there just perfectly.

The pressure you apply with your fingers should be steady and deep enough to meet some resistance, but not so deep it causes more than a pleasurable pain. Just hang there with that pressure for about 30 seconds, remembering to feel that your shoulders are relaxed, and remembering to

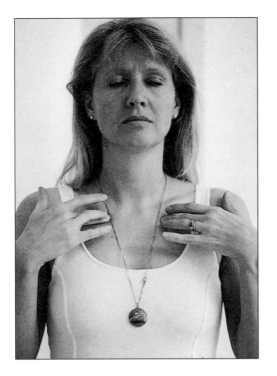

These points help to balance the analytical and intuitive functions of the brain.

keep breathing. You'll feel yourself settling a bit, centring, and you might even notice that your vision seems to clear. It's also good for headaches, irritability and head colds. The "gates of consciousness"... has a nice sound to it, mm?

ON THE RIGHT, our model is showing another set of shiatsu points, these to help balance the functions of the left and right brain. The points lie in the little hollows you'll find if you explore with your fingers, just underneath the collarbone, a little to the inside of a line drawn straight down from the outside edges of the neck. These "brain buttons" will help you get yourself out of being in just one side of your head, and back into a more balanced view of what's in front of you.

Here's a variety of things you can do to give yourself a fresh start whenever you need one throughout the day. They're simple, mostly unobtrusive, and you can do them no matter what shape you're in. The only real effort you have to make is to remember to do them! Sneak them into your list of "to-do's". Programme the alarm on your computer to beep you every 40 minutes or so – time for a break!

Ten 30-Second Holidays
for Desk Jockeys

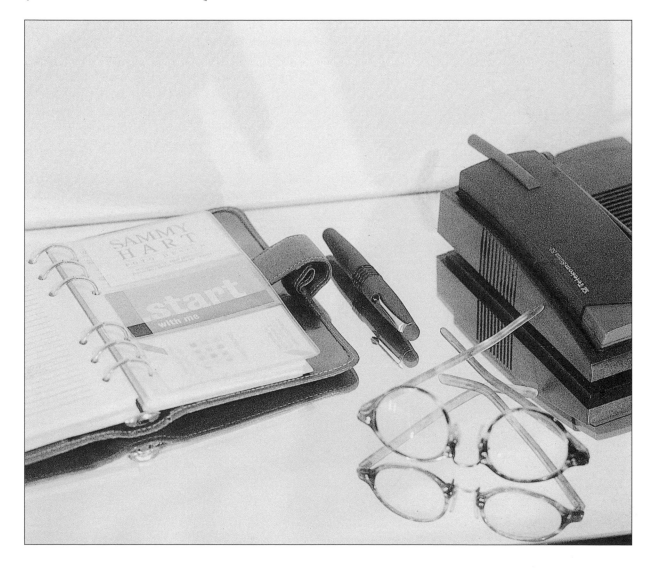

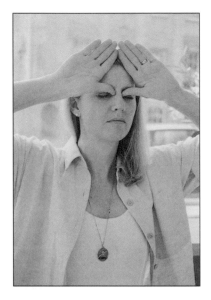

1 THE PHOTOGRAPH ON the left is just to show you how the hands should be placed in relation to the forehead in the photo below. We don't actually expect you to make this gesture in the middle of the office – if you did, your colleagues would be certain to think your body had been occupied by a Zombie from Galaxy B29X47!

Placing your hands in this way on your forehead does two things: one, it gives you a nice comfortable cushion to rest your head on, and two it tends to help you slip more easily into that "meditation" space we were talking about earlier.

Clear off enough space so that your elbows can rest on the desk, and as you relax into your little holiday, let your awareness rest just there in the forehead, in the diamond shape made by your hands. Take a deep breath, and as you let it go bring even more awareness to that space. Don't forget to come back....

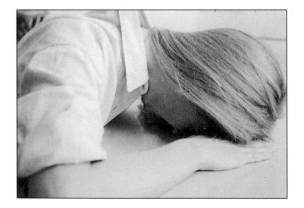

2 THESE POINTS ARE in the middle of that big muscle that runs across the back of the shoulders, and they're easy to find because they always hurt! When you're about to get a tension headache, or your neck feels like it's turned to a pillar of salt, or your hands have started to numb from the effort to hold yourself together, these points are good. If you've stored up a lot of unexpressed emotions, though, you might find that they want to come out – so go easy at first, and if it's not a safe environment to "let go" then you might want to wait until you get home. When you've located the points, keep the pressure deep and steady, feeling the tension that's hiding in there beginning to dissolve and let go. You can prop your elbows up on your desk for support.

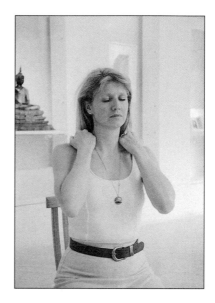

3 DON'T EXPECT YOURSELF to be able to touch your hands together behind your back immediately like our model in this photo, and don't think there's anything wrong if you can't. However close together you can manage to get the hands without straining is fine, and will help your neck and shoulders to relax. First one hand above and then the other, to balance both sides – and you will probably notice that there is some difference in flexibility between one arm and the other. As you do it more, you'll find your flexibility increases on its own, without needing you to force it.

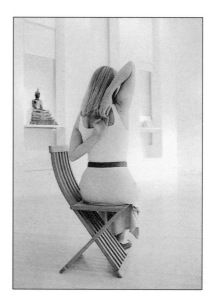

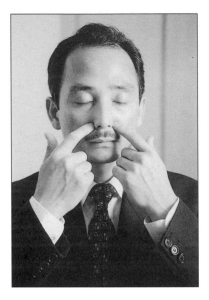

4 MOST OF US will go to work when we have a cold, hay fever, or a stuffy nose. But it's not much fun, and our brains don't seem to work very well when we're in this state. These points right at the corners of the nostrils help to clear the nose and sinuses, and can air out that stuffy feeling in the head. The points also assist in relaxing the face muscles generally.

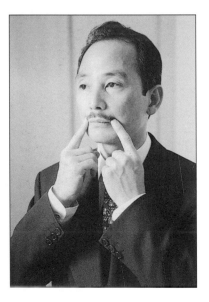

5 YOU CAN FIND these points by drawing an imaginary line straight down from your pupils as you look straight ahead, and just in line with the corners of your mouth. It's nice to do when you've been smiling without feeling a smile, or clenching your teeth, or otherwise "holding yourself together" in a way that has created tension all over, particularly in the face. Just hold the spots for about 30 seconds, closing your eyes if you can and putting your awareness on the place where the fingertips meet the skin.

6 IT'S AMAZING HOW refreshing and relaxing this tiny little movement of the ears can be. Very gently, take the tops of both ears between thumb and index finger, and just curve them around towards the front. Hold them there for just a few moments. If you like, you can – again, very gently – pull them slightly away from the head. You'll find yourself wanting to take a nice deep breath, and as you let it go all kinds of tensions will just wash away, like standing under a shower of relaxation that moves from your head down through your body.

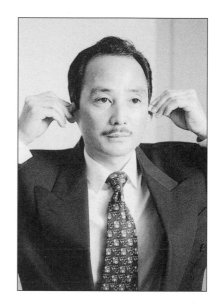

7 UNLESS YOU HAVE a specific back problem that prevents you from doing this simple twist, it really can't be done too often. Put your feet flat on the floor, and grasp the back of your chair with one hand, pulling yourself gently around and turning your head to look behind you at the same time. Twist first to one side, and then to the other, taking care not to strain or push – you don't get any extra points for making a 180 degree turn. Also, take care that you're keeping your shoulders relaxed and breathing naturally as you do it. When you get back to work, your posture will be better and your spine will have let go of a lot of tension.

One interesting variation on this exercise is to first do it as shown, letting your head follow the movement of your torso. Then, repeat the twisting motion but this time keep your head facing forward. You won't be able to twist as far, of course. But for some reason, if you then repeat the first movement, you'll find that you can actually see farther behind you than before.

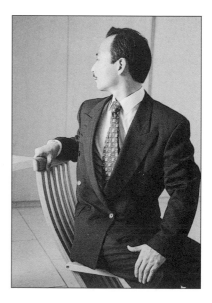

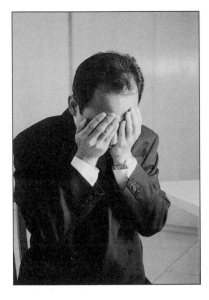

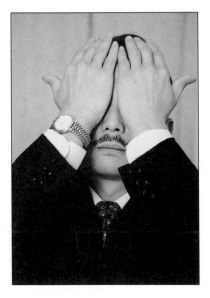

8 IF YOU GET very good at this one, you can prolong it and have a little nap! Just put your elbows on the desk, and put your face in your hands, cupping your palms over your eyes as shown so that your face can be supported without being "poked" uncomfortably anywhere. Relax your shoulders, and sink into that soft, welcoming darkness for a few moments. Hopefully none of your colleagues will come rushing over to ask you what's the matter – prop the book up on your desk, so they can see that you're doing "an exercise" and not just goofing off. Call up a specially created page on your computer screen that says in big letters, RELAXING – DO NOT DISTURB. Even if you can just manage ten seconds, you'll feel like you've gone home for a nap.

9 MANY PEOPLE HAVE the misconception that Tantra is all about sex – it is not. There are many, many small exercises and meditations that come from the Tantra tradition and the purpose of all of them is to help us find that relaxed, thought-less space of meditation. This one is easy to do, almost anywhere, and you can either do it for just a few moments to refresh yourself or go into it deeply, as a meditation. What follows is Osho's commentary on the technique as it appears in the classic Tantra text, *Vigyan Bhairav Tantra.*

Touching eyeballs as a feather,
Lightness between them opens into heart
And there permeates the cosmos.

Touching eyeballs as a feather... Use both your palms, put them on your eyes, and allow the palms to touch the eyeballs – but just like a feather, with no pressure. If you press you miss the point, you miss the whole technique. Don't press; just touch like a feather. You will have to adjust, because in the beginning you will be pressing. Put less and less pressure until you are just touching with no pressure at all — just your palms touch the eyeballs. Just a touch, just a meeting with no pressure, because if the pressure is there, then the technique will not function. So – *like a feather.*

Why? Because a needle can do something which a sword cannot do. If you press, the quality of touch has changed — you are aggressive. And the energy that is flowing through the eyes is very subtle: a small pressure and it starts fighting and a resistance is created. If you press, then the energy that is flowing through the eyes will start a resistance, a fight; a struggle will ensue. So don't press; even a slight pressure is enough for the eye energy to judge.

It is very subtle, it is very delicate. Don't press — like a feather, just your palm is touching, as if not touching. Touching as if not touching, no pressure; just a touch, a slight feeling that the palm is touching the eyeball, that's all.

What will happen? When you simply touch without any pressure, the energy starts moving within. If you press, it starts fighting with the hand, with the palm, and moves out. Just a touch and the energy starts moving within. The door is closed; simply the door is closed and the energy falls back. The moment energy falls back, you will feel a lightness coming all over your face, your head. This energy moving back makes you light.

And just between these two eyes is the third eye, the wisdom eye, the prajna-chakshu. Just between these two eyes is the third eye. The energy falling back from the eyes hits the third eye. That's why one feels light, levitating, as if there is no gravitation. And from the third eye the energy falls on the heart. It is a physical process: just drip, drip, it drops, and you will feel a very light feeling entering in your heart. The heartbeats will slow down, the breathing will slow down. Your whole body will feel relaxed.

Even if you are not entering deep meditation, this will help you physically. Any time in the day, relax on a chair – or if you don't have any chair, when just sitting in a train – close your eyes, feel a relaxed being in the whole of your body, and then put both your palms on your eyes. But don't press – that's the very significant thing. Just touch *like a feather.*

When you touch and don't press, your thoughts will stop immediately. In a relaxed mind thoughts cannot move; they get frozen. They need frenzy and fever, they need tension to move. They live through tension. When the eyes are silent, relaxed, and the energy is moving backwards, thoughts will stop. You will feel a certain quality of euphoria, and that will deepen daily.

So do it many times in the day. Even for a single moment, touching will be good. Whenever your eyes feel exhausted, dry of energy, exploited – after reading, seeing a film, or watching TV – whenever you feel it, just close the eyes and touch. Immediately there will be the effect. But if you want to make it a meditation, then do it for at least 40 minutes. And the whole thing is not to press.

Because it is easy for a single moment to have a feather-like touch; it is difficult for 40 minutes. Many times you will forget and you will start pressing.

Don't press. For 40 minutes, just remain aware that your hands have no weight; they are just touching. Continue being aware that you are not pressing, only touching. This will become a deep awareness, just like breathing. As Buddha says to breathe with full awareness, the same will happen with touching, because you have to be constantly mindful that you are not pressing. Your hand should just be a feather, a weightless thing, simply touching.

Your mind will be totally there, alert, near the eyes, and the energy will be flowing constantly. In the beginning it will be just dropping in drops. Within months you will feel it has become a river-like thing, and within a year you will feel it has become a flood. And when it happens – touching eyeballs as a feather, lightness between them – when you touch you will feel lightness. You can feel it right now. Immediately, the moment you touch, a lightness comes. And that lightness between them opens into the heart; that lightness penetrates, opens into the heart. In the heart, only lightness can enter; nothing heavy can enter. Only very light things can happen to the heart.

This lightness between the two eyes will start dropping into the heart, and the heart will open to receive it – and there permeates the cosmos. As the falling energy becomes a stream and then a river and then a flood, you will be washed completely, washed away. You will not feel that you are. You will feel simply the cosmos is. Breathing in, breathing out, you will feel you have become the cosmos. The cosmos comes in and the cosmos goes out. The entity that you have always been, the ego, will not be there.

This technique is very simple, without any danger, so you can experiment with it as you like. But because it is so easy, you may not be able to do it. The whole thing depends on touch without pressure, so you will have to learn it. Try it. Within a week it will happen. Suddenly some day when you are just touching with no pressure, immediately you will feel what I am saying – a lightness and an opening in the heart, and something dropping from the head into the heart.[19]

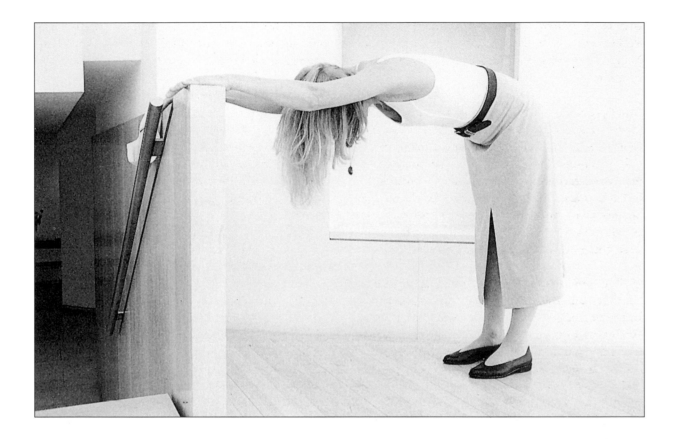

10 THIS LAST EXERCISE is great for opening and relaxing the whole spine, and when you do it you'll also feel a pleasant, circulation-enhancing stretch in the back of the legs, too. Get a good grip on the table, and stand far enough away from it so you can bend at a 90 degree angle. Once you're in position, use your awareness to help you let go of the tension in your shoulders, relaxing them more and more, bit by bit. If you keep your spine straight as you do this, it will begin to sink down between the shoulder blades until it feels like your whole spine is just hanging there like a bridge between your shoulder blades and your hip bones. Take care to keep the head down and not to let the lower back cave in. You might be tempted to bounce, but that's not such a good idea. When it feels like time to straighten up again, take it slow and easy.

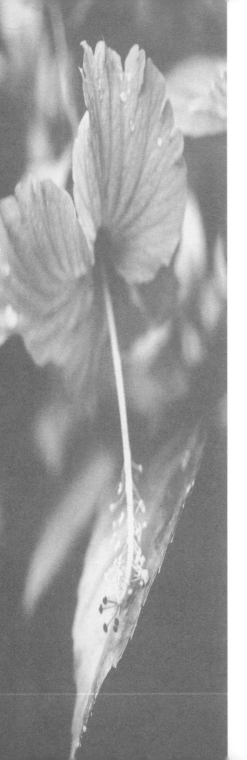

It's mid-morning, and you feel like you've already put in a full day's work. Or, you've just finished a troublesome task and you want to give yourself a little reward. Or, you're stuck on a problem and feel like you need a jump-start.

WAIT! Before you grab that cup and fill your tank with more coffee, try one of the drug-free pick-me-ups on the following pages. They'll give you the same kind of wake-up call but without the jangle of nerves and the disturbance of tummy.

Afterwards, if you still really want that cup of coffee or tea, then go ahead – but with just a few small changes. Make it a ceremony, a real treat for yourself. Prepare it just the way you like it, enjoying the fragrance, being aware of the texture of the cup. (You wouldn't drink that vending-machine coffee, would you??!) Sip it slowly, savouring the taste, feeling the buzz that comes to your body after you've swallowed it. Take the time just to drink it, not doing anything else. When you've had enough, toss out the rest of it. Now, you can get back to work!

Caffeine-free Pick-Me-Ups

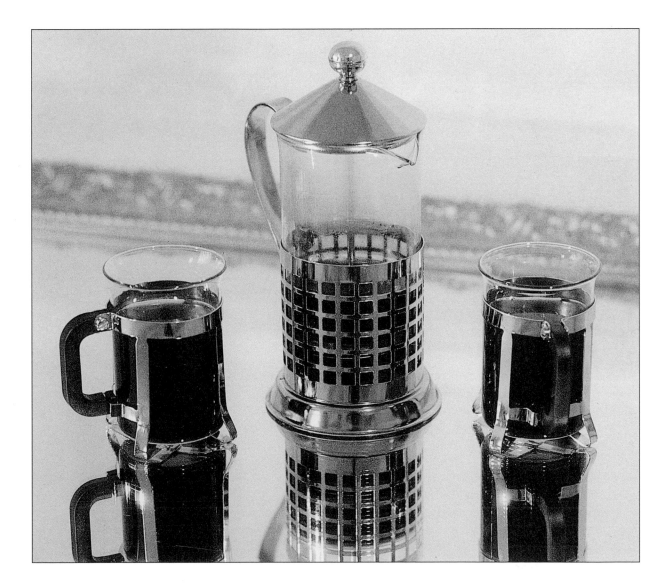

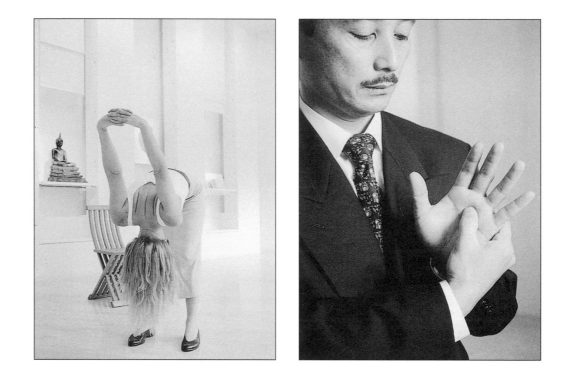

1 You might remember this one from the morning exercises. It's included here again because it works in no time at all to give the body a good allover stretch and get the circulation moving after you've been sitting so long at your desk that you're beginning to feel more like a robot than a human being. Clasp your hands behind your back, palms up. Inhale deeply, and then bend forward as you exhale, letting your head hang loose and reaching up towards the ceiling with your clasped hands. Go slowly on the way down, so you don't lose your balance, and slowly come back up too, so you don't get dizzy.

2 This shiatsu point on the palm of your hand is good for times when you feel really exhausted but have to carry on. The point lies between the spot where the middle and ring fingers rest on the palm of the hand. You'll feel the little

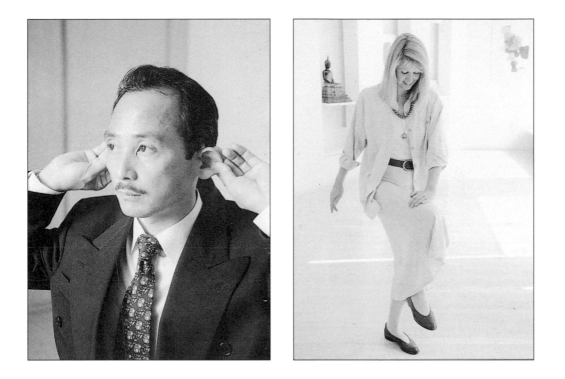

groove between two bones, and that's where it is. Once you've found it, just hold it firmly or masssage it, for up to two minutes.

3 This is easy to do and, like the exercise on the previous page, it doesn't require you to get up from your desk. Give both ears a gentle but thorough massage, starting from the bottom and pulling out gently as you go.

4 Sometimes we can get tired and sleepy just by using the brain too much in one hemisphere. Whether we're doing mathematics or trying to think up a new advertising campaign, our poor brains can get a bit lopsided and groggy in the process. This exercise is so much fun, and so silly-looking, you'll have to enlist everybody's participation if you're in an open-plan office! It's simple: just march in place, raising your knees up high and

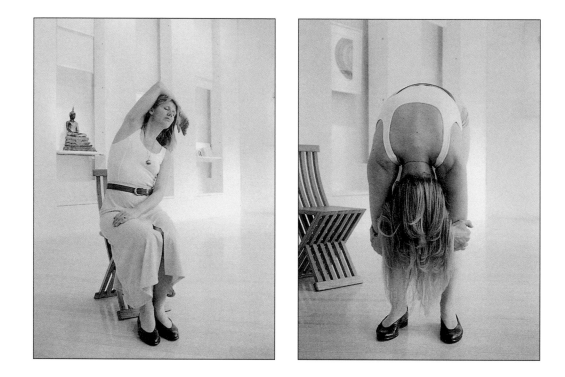

slapping each raised knee with the palm of the opposite hand. Left ... left ... left-right-left. Got it? It's balancing out the left and right hemispheres of the brain, at the same time it's getting you up and moving!

5/6 These simple stretches will help relieve the stiffness that comes from sitting too long in one position. In the first, rest one arm across the top of your head, with the other lying loose in your lap. Let the weight of the arm push you – gently! – to one side, taking care to avoid twisting the back. Then change the position of the arms and stretch the other side. It's good to follow this one by standing up, crossing both arms across the top of your head and leaning over, just hanging out there for a few moments and letting your back stretch out and your shoulders and arms relax. Keep your knees a bit flexed so you don't fall over.

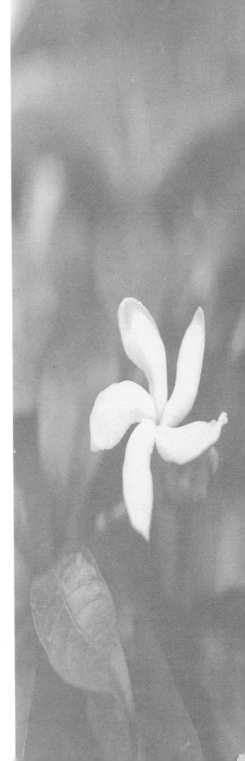

"We are so tense, not only because there are circumstances which make us tense, but basically we have completely forgotten how to relax. So if even if there are no circumstances to make you tense, you will still be tense. We are tense. We have forgotten completely relaxation, the art of let-go.

This must be taught. Relaxation is the language which is not being taught – that is the forgotten language. The whole of education, the whole of society is teaching everybody to be tense."[20]

Unwind...Before You Unravel!

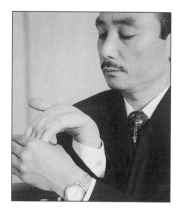

AS ENERGY CIRCULATES in the body, it can get trapped in the places where we are tense — especially in the joints near the extremities. This in turn can affect the whole flow of energy in the body, causing us to feel "all wound up" like a too-tight spring. Here are a few things you can do throughout the day, whenever you think of them, to unsnarl the traffic jam of tensions in your ankles and wrists, and to unwind your whole bodymind system in the process.

1/2 You can prop your elbows up on the desk to do this exercise, to make it easier. Just let the weight of one hand pull the other one down, first forward and then backward as shown by our model here. As you breathe out, let the wrists and the hands relax even more. Don't force anything, and be careful not to actually pull down on the

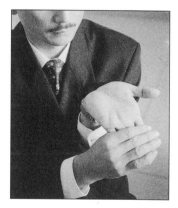

hand. If you just let the whole exercise be loose, the pressure on the wrists will be just the right amount. This exercise, and the following one, are especially good for those who spend lots of time typing on a keyboard.

3/4 This is a very gentle movement, and if you are normally pretty flexible you might not "feel" it much at all. The real benefit comes from the actual dance of the movement itself, which is uncommon enough that the brain sits up and takes notice, and helps to spread the relaxation of it throughout the rest of the body. Grasp one hand with the other as shown in picture 3. Now, use that hand to turn the other to the second position, as shown in picture 4. Start the movement with the hands placed at the level of the upper chest, and as you do the turning motion, bring

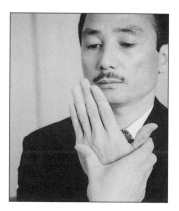

both hands down to the place just below the navel. This helps to keep you from straining the muscles, or pulling them in the wrong way, and also assist you so that you become able to "centre" your energy.

5/6 This is better for you than jiggling your foot. Jiggling your foot is your body's effort to get rid of tension, but because it's so unconscious and habitual with so many people, it can actually set up a cycle of even greater tension. So reset the computer inside your brain and get it to remind you – next time you're sitting there with your legs crossed and find yourself jiggling your foot, change gears. Stop going up and down, and go in circles instead, slow and large circles, first one direction and then the other. Keep doing it until the movement smoothes out. Then re-cross your legs and let the other foot have its share of the fun!

A man of awareness simply slips from one moment to another, just like a dewdrop slipping from the blade of grass, not carrying anything. A man of awareness has no cargo, he moves unburdened. Then everything is new, and then no problems are created.[21]

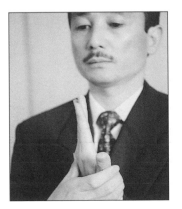

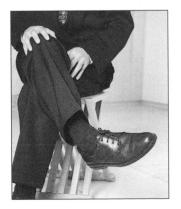

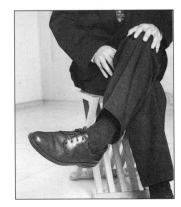

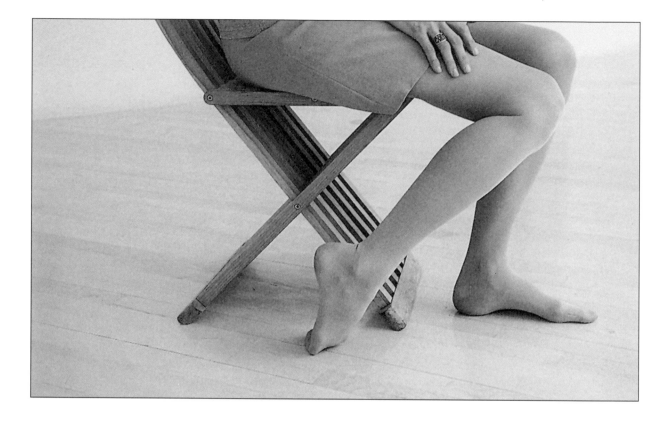

7 You'll have to slip out of your shoes to do this ... women who wear heels will appreciate the opportunity! If you have an adjustable chair, you might want to raise it a bit, or lower it, so your foot can rest comfortably on the floor. You can feel free to experiment a little, just as long as you keep your attention with the movements and don't get distracted. When you're distracted, wrong moves can happen and cause a cramp in your foot. It won't damage you, but it can be pretty uncomfortable! Using your natural weight, without extra pressure, bend the toes forward and backward, and rotate them around. The point is to give your feet a good "cat stretch."

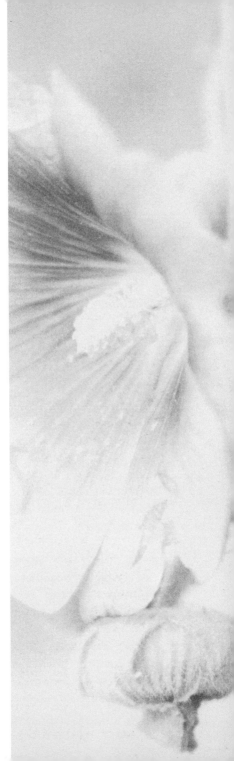

"Awareness is needed, not condemnation – and through awareness transformation happens spontaneously. If you become aware of your anger, understanding penetrates. Just watching, with no judgment, not saying good, not saying bad, just watching in your inner sky. There is lightning, anger, you feel hot, the whole nervous system shaking and quaking, and you feel a tremor all over the body – a beautiful moment, because when energy functions you can watch it easily; when it is not functioning you cannot watch.

Close your eyes and meditate on it. Don't fight, just look at what is happening. The whole sky filled with electricity, so much lightning, so much beauty – just lie down on the ground and look at the sky and watch. Then do the same inside."[22]

If You Can't Freak Out, Freak In

QUITE A LOT of our tension is related to emotions that come up during the day which, because of a variety of circumstances, we feel we can't express. When we get angry, for example, it's not just a mind thing – the breathing changes, the body heats up or twists itself into knots. When we feel afraid or "nervous" then again the breathing changes, the heart beats faster and we get "butterflies" in the stomach. If we have to pretend on the surface that everything is just fine, then we suppress these bodily reactions. If this kind of behavior goes on over a long time, we can develop serious diseases.

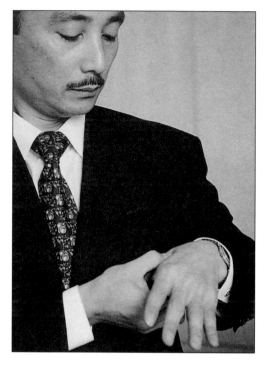

This point between thumb and forefinger is good for centring, and very effective in relieving tension headaches.

chance to express itself in a non-harmful, safe way. Emotions, if we can accept them as natural, without judging them to be "good" or "bad," are notoriously transient. We can do a lot to help them along their way if we do just a few simple things to give our bodies a chance to shake them off as they arise. If we can relieve the body of the memory of its hurt or fear or anger, then it's just a short step to being able to let go of the emotion on the mental level, too. Soon the day comes when we find – often to our own surprise – that we are no longer so affected by others as we used to be. When that happens, we have really learned how not to freak out, but to "freak in" – to be so centred and at home in

"Swallowing" our emotions can contribute to stomach ulcers. Not being able to express our anger, to "get it off our chests" can set the stage for a heart attack. Living with the feeling that somebody is always "on your back" can result in chronic back pain. "Sitting on" your feelings can cause troubles with the bowels and colon. The exercises in this section are small things you can do to let off steam during the day, to give your body a

ourselves that the transient disturbances of everyday life become just one more opportunity to watch the ever-changing movie of our lives.

The watching of our emotions comes later, though. First, try these simple physical things to give your body a break from all the tensions it encounters day by day. Let it know you're not going to ignore its needs anymore. The rest of the changes will soon start to happen by themselves.

PICTURED OPPOSITE PAGE:
On the web of the hand between thumb and index finger of the left hand, there's a shiatsu point which is actually quite useful for relieving tension headaches. You can find it easily, because it's almost always quite tender, and it is located just at the v-shaped junction of two of the bones in your hand. This point is good when you need to "collect" yourself in a generally tense and chaotic situation, when you're just about to freak out because everything seems all too much at once, when you find yourself snapping at your colleagues or your family because you've just got too many things on your mind.

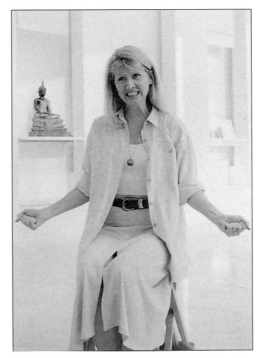

Clenching your fists gives the body an outlet for its "fight or flight" responses, and gives you a safe outlet for anger or frustration.

Just hold the point, using the thumb and index finger of the right hand to create a firm pressure. As you hold the point, become aware of your breathing and let it relax if it is irregular or disturbed. Close your eyes, if you can. But if you can't – if you're sitting in the middle of one of those meetings where everybody is interrupting everybody else, for example, it's okay. Just settle inside yourself for a minute or two, and rest there while the storm rages on around you.

PHOTO THIS PAGE:
Whenever you feel irritated, angry, frustrated, it's a wonderful release just to clench and unclench your fists several times. You can hide them under the table if necessary... but do it! Not only will it help to keep your body healthy and alive rather than repressed and confused – you'll soon find that the anger itself begins to cool down when you give it this simple, physical outlet.

> If you want to beat someone, beat the empty sky. If you want to be angry, be angry; if you want to scream, scream. But do it alone, and remember yourself as a point which is seeing all this, this drama. Then it becomes a psychodrama, and you can laugh at it and it will be a deep catharsis for you.

Afterwards you will feel relieved of it – and not only relieved of it, you will have gained something through it. You will have matured; a growth will have come to you. And now you will know that even while you were in anger there was a within which was undisturbed.[23]

"THE MOMENT THE other is there, you are less concerned about yourself; you are more concerned about what his opinion will be about you. When you are alone in your bathroom, you become almost like a child — sometimes you make faces before the mirror. But if you become suddenly aware that even a small child is looking through the keyhole, you immediately change: you become your ordinary, old self again — serious, sober, as people expect you to be.

And the most amazing thing is that you are afraid of those people and they are afraid of you — everybody is afraid of everybody else. Nobody is allowing his feelings, his reality, his authenticity — but everybody wants to do it, because it is a very suicidal act to go on repressing your original face.

You are not living; on the contrary you are simply acting. And because the whole world is watching, your centuries-long unconscious holds you back — not to express, not to come out of the mask of your personality. Everybody is hiding behind something false — it hurts. To be dishonest, to be insincere to yourself, is the worst punishment you can give to yourself.... And in fact, who cares? Perhaps people will think, once, that you are a little crazy — at the most — and once they have accepted that you are a little crazy, then there is nothing to fear. And what is wrong in being called crazy? The world has known such beautiful, crazy people... in fact, all the great people in the world have been a little bit crazy — crazy in the eyes of the crowd. They were living each moment with totality and intensity, and because of this totality and intensity, their life became a beautiful flower — they were full of fragrance, love and life and laughter.[24]"

THE LAST EXERCISE in this section is good for all kinds of "freaking in." Maybe you're so happy you can't contain it, or so sad you're afraid you'll break down and start crying right in the middle of the office. Maybe you've just come out of a three-hour ordeal with the most arrogant man you have ever met, and because he's your most important client you had to smile and shake his hand at the end. Quick, before you do anything else, go find someplace where you can be alone — preferably with a mirror — and let your face express everything you can't possibly ever, ever say with words. For a little encouragement and inspiration, on this page are a few words from Osho on the subject of faces, original and pretended.

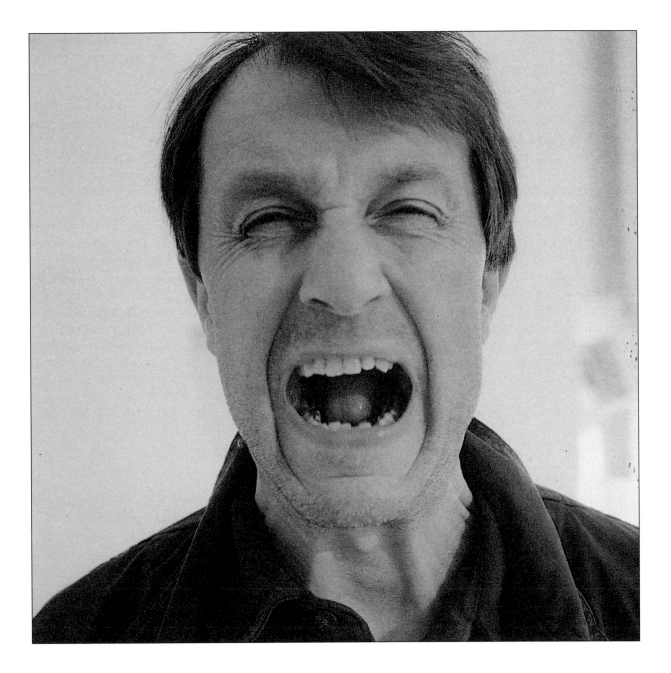

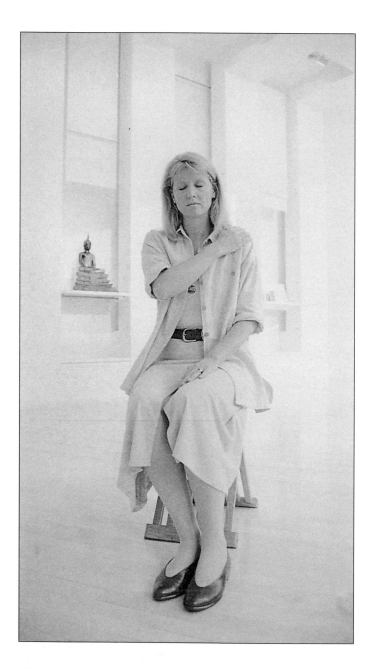

ANOTHER REMINDER about the breath ... and a good technique for relaxing those places in the body where we can actually feel the tension in the form of discomfort or pain. When you realize you've been hunched up at your desk clutching the phone for the past two hours and now your shoulder hurts, take a few moments to consciously relax. Close your eyes, put your hand on your shoulder to help you to direct your attention there, and breathe. Breathe in — and direct the breath to the shoulder, or whatever part of the body that is feeling tense right now. As you breathe out, let the breath go out through that tense part of the body, soothing and creating space inside the muscles, allowing the tightness to dissolve, relaxing, letting go. Again — breathe in, directing the breath to the tension in the body. Breathe out, and let the breath take the tension away, dissolving it and dispersing it as it goes.

"Life consists of sipping a cup of tea, of gossiping with a friend; going for a morning walk, not going anywhere in particular, just for a walk, no goal, no end, from any point you can turn back; cooking food for someone you love; cooking food for yourself, because you love your body too; washing your clothes, cleaning the floor, watering the garden... these small things, very small things...."[25]

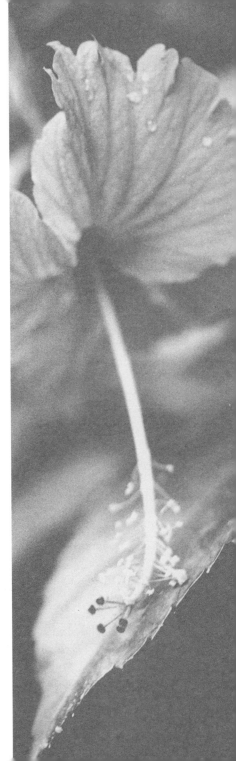

EveryBody's Home Companion

" A DISCIPLE HAD come to see Ikkyu, his master. The disciple had been practising for some time. It was raining, and as he went in, he left his shoes and umbrella outside. After he paid his respects, the master asked him on which side of his shoes he had left his umbrella.

Now, what kind of question...? You don't expect masters to ask such nonsense questions – you expect them to ask about God, about kundalini rising, chakras opening, lights happening in your head. You ask questions about such great things – the occult, the esoteric.

But Ikkyu asked a very ordinary question. No Christian saint would have asked it, no Jain monk would have asked it, no Hindu swami would have asked it. It can be done only by one who is really with the Buddha, *in* the Buddha – who is really a Buddha. The master asked him on which side of his shoes he had left his umbrella. Now, what do shoes and umbrellas have to do with spirituality?

If the same question was asked to you, you would have felt annoyed. You would have felt that this man is no master at all. What kind of question is this? What philosophy can there be in it?

But there is something immensely valuable in it. Had he asked about God, about your kundalini and chakras, that would have been nonsense, utterly meaningless. But this has meaning. The disciple could not remember – who bothers where you have put your shoes and on which side you have put your umbrella, to the right or to the left. Who bothers? Who pays so much attention to umbrellas? Who thinks of shoes? Who is so careful?

But that was enough – the disciple was refused. Ikkyu said, "Then go and meditate for seven years more."

"Seven years?" the disciple said. "Just for this small fault?"

Ikkyu said, "This is not a small fault. Faults are not small or big – you are just not yet living meditatively, that's all. Go back, meditate for seven years more, and come again."

This is the essential message of Buddhism: be careful, careful of everything. And don't make any distinction between things – that this is trivia and that is very, very spiritual. It depends on you. Pay attention, be careful, and everything becomes spiritual. Don't pay attention, don't be careful, and everything becomes unspiritual.

Spirituality is imparted by you, it is your gift to the world. When a master like Ikkyu touches his umbrella, the umbrella is as divine as anything can be – and if you touch even god, god will become trivia. It depends on your touch.

Meditative energy is alchemical. It transforms the base metal into gold; it goes on transforming the baser into the higher. The more meditative you become, the more you see god everywhere. At the ultimate peak, everything is divine. This very world is the paradise, and this very body the Buddha.[26] "

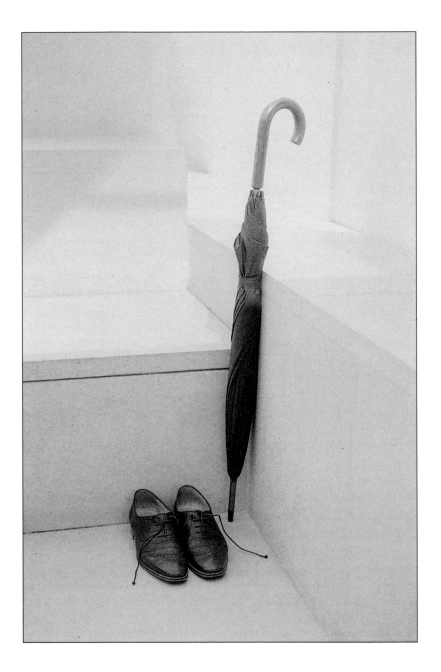

Get Yourself a New Attitude

ZEN MASTERS LIKE Ikkyu are renowned for their reverence for the small things of life. "What did you do before your enlightenment?" they are asked, and they say, "I chopped wood, I carried water from the well."

"And what do you do now that you are enlightened?" they are asked. "I chop wood, I carry water from the well," is their reply.

Of course, the woodchopping and the watercarrying have a totally different quality when they are done with the clarity and awareness of one who is enlightened. Each small act is an act of meditation. Chopping wood, placing the shoes next to the umbrella, cleaning rice, sweeping the floor – no activity is too lowly or too unimportant to be done unconsciously, robot-like, unaware. In fact, it is much easier to be aware when we are doing simple physical activities. Our minds are not really required, so there's no distraction of thoughts, and our bodies have performed these tasks hundreds of times, so there's no tension of trying to learn how to do something new. Relaxed, thoughtless, the only thing left to do

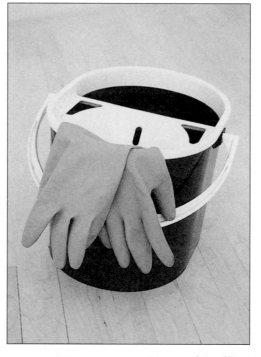

is to be simply alert to the movements of the body, present to the sensations of the body. Right?

Well, not exactly. Not for most of us, anyway – most of us squander these opportunities for meditation and relaxation by trying to finish things as quickly as possible so we can go out and "have a good time." It's no surprise that most accidents happen in the home. While people are at home, doing the small chores of cleaning and maintenance around the house, their minds are a thousand miles or many hours away, planning what they're going to do once this onerous task is over. And when we aren't "present" to what we are doing, that's when we fall off ladders and nail our own thumbs to the wall.

Somewhere along the way, we seem to have acquired the idea that simple activities like cleaning, doing the laundry, washing the dishes, are "chores." Even the very word sounds like something you don't want to do – something you have to be bribed into doing with a weekly allowance, perhaps?

And now you're a grown-up, you don't even have that reward to look forward to.

Just as an experiment, try spending your next day around the house simply doing whatever needs to be done. No need to be thinking about what comes next – it will come when it comes, and your thinking about it will only make you inattentive and inefficient in the present moment – "Now, what have I done with that screwdriver?" Be alert for opportunities to have fun – sing to the vacuum cleaner or have a little dance with the broom. Experiment with using your senses in a new way – admire the shiny chrome of the faucet with your eyes, feel the texture of the laundry with your hands, play with the soap bubbles in the sink and listen to the little popping sounds they make, give yourself a good stretch by getting down on your hands and knees to clean the floor.

There's nothing wrong with housework. In fact, for those of us who work with our heads all the time it can really be a wonderfully refreshing change. Get yourself a new attitude – and in the process, find a new way to relax and let your tensions fall away.

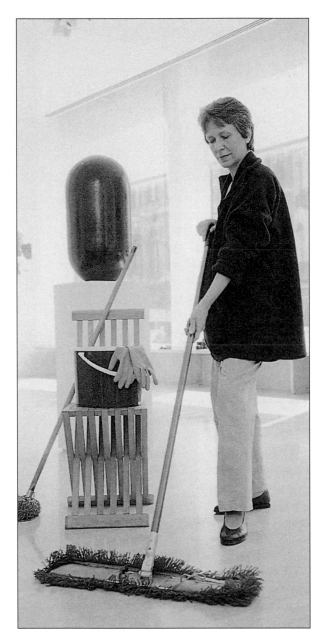

Deprogramming the Robot

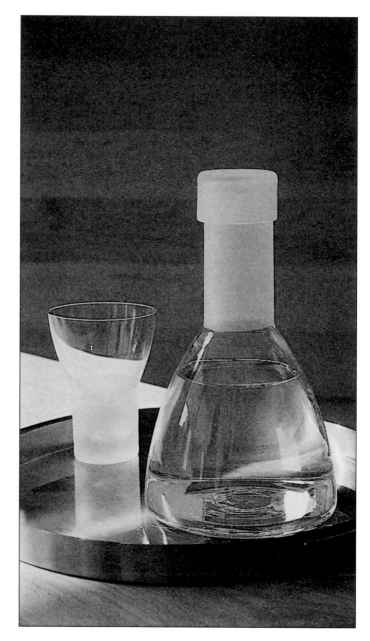

ONE OF THE best ways to start being alert about the little everyday things you do is to experiment with doing them differently. It's like learning to drive a car – when you first get behind the wheel, you're aware of every little movement you make. The very newness of the situation requires your total attention. Once you've learned, though, all those small movements get taken over by the robot in your brain. You don't have to think about them, so your mind is free to wander off in other directions.

The problem for the body when we function in robot mode, is that it has trouble getting our attention when it wants us to change what we're doing. Robots are notoriously dense when it comes to interpreting subtle signals that go against the programme. So while it's true that you might not notice dramatic improvements in your physical condition if you start tying your shoelaces with awareness, by doing so you will be providing the soil for your awareness to grow. And as your awareness grows, you live less in the future and in the past, more in the present moment. As you live more in the

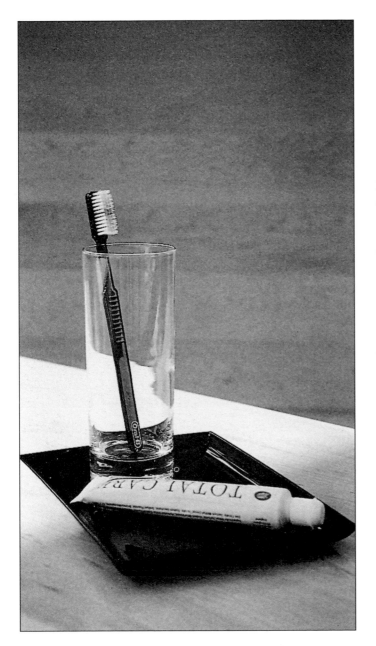

present moment, you become more relaxed. And as you become more relaxed, you become more receptive to your body's own natural wisdom and start functioning according to it, not according to the robot.

Start with something simple, like brushing your teeth. Use the hand opposite to the one you normally use. Slows you down, doesn't it? And makes you aware of the smallest things – how the bristles of the toothbrush feel against your gums, whether or not you have actually covered all the little nooks and crannies of your mouth. You might not remember it now, but this is how it felt when you first started learning to brush your teeth. Try it again and again, every few days. See what you can re-learn about brushing your teeth by using this simple device. Then look for other opportunities – getting dressed, putting on your shoes, carrying your bag or briefcase, using the telephone. If you look, you'll find dozens of small tasks that will give you a chance to experiment with deprogramming the robot and making more space for awareness and spontaneity in your life.

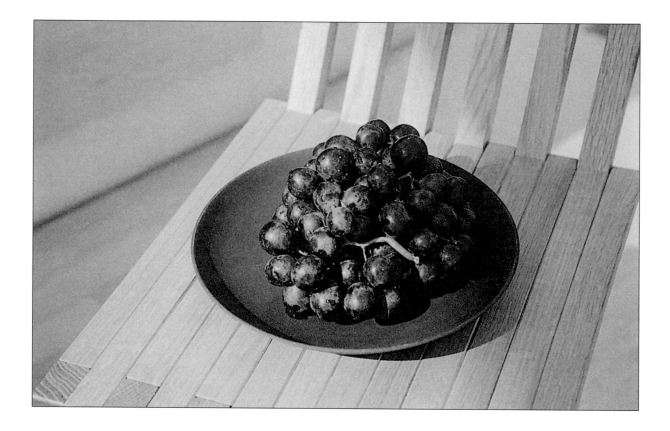

You Are How You Eat

WHILE WE'RE ON the subject of robotic behaviour…

Everybody's talking about food these days. How much of it to eat, what kinds of it, how much cholesterol, how much fibre, how many pesticides, hormones or antibiotics it might contain, and whether it's junk, fast, or ready for the microwave. No, we are not going to launch into a set of recommendations about what you should eat. Instead, we're going to suggest you have a look at how you eat. Once you sort out the how, the what will tend to take care of itself very nicely.

To keep it as simple as possible, start with this exercise:

Go into your kitchen and have a look at what's there to eat, leaving aside all the herbs and spices and condiments and so on. Get a piece of paper and something to write with, and make three columns. The categories are not necessarily mutually exclusive, so as you make your lists under them feel free to put an item in more than one column.

The heading at the top of the first column is "convenience." You have this food in your kitchen because it's not much trouble to prepare, or you can eat it straight out of the bag, or you can give it to the kids when they complain about being hungry. This column doesn't have to be exclusively "junk food" or frozen dinners. It can be fruits and vegetables too, if you have the knack of preparing them without making a big fuss about it.

The heading at the top of the second is "body." Your body appreciates this food, feels better after you've eaten it, whispers in your ear that it's good for you. Take some time to really "feel" what's true before you put an item in this column, and don't confuse it with "taste." You might like the taste of chocolate, for example, but maybe it upsets your stomach when you eat it. Or, you might not be so crazy about the taste of olives but sometimes your body just craves them, and nothing else will do. What we're looking for here in this column is what Leonard Pearson has called "humming food," food that sends all the cells in your body into celebration when you eat it. The same food might not "hum" with you every day, day in, day out. But the reason you have it around is because basically, your body loves it.

The third column is headed with the word "mind." What do we mean by this? This is for the category of food that you have because the kids have seen it on television and demanded it. Or, because you like the taste of it even though every cell in your body tells you it's no good for you. It's the food you have because you like the way the package looks, but otherwise can't imagine why you've bought it. It's what you eat when you're restless, or bored, or sitting in front of the television and you're not even sure what it tastes like or whether your body likes it because you've never taken any notice. It's also what you have around because you've been told it's "good for you" but actually you can't stand the taste and haven't noticed that it makes you feel in any way more nourished or healthier.

If you've had trouble with this exercise, that's a great start! You're on the road to being more aware of not just what, but how you eat.

The second part of the exercise is to take the question marks and look into them, one at a time, for the coming week. The next time you open the bag of potato chips, take the first one out slowly. Stop doing whatever else it is that you're doing, and put the potato chip in your mouth. Taste it, feel the texture of it, feel what it does to your tongue. Chew it, swallow it, feel it as it travels down to your stomach. If you don't like it, does it mean you should give up potato chips? Maybe, maybe not. Maybe you just need to find a different brand, one that "hums" something a little closer to your tune. Or, maybe you weren't sure about the courgette. They're always available in the market, and they're easy to cook, so they're convenient, but does your body really like them? Pay attention the next time you prepare them, feel the texture and smell the fragrance of them. If you always cook them, cut a little slice and eat it raw. If you like it, it becomes even more convenient, and if you can find a ready-made dip to go with it, it's a good substitute for the potato chips. After you cook them, take time to really taste them and feel how your body responds. Are you spicing them too much, or not enough? Could you cook them a little less, preserving more of the freshness, and enjoy them more?

The point is to take the time to become more aware when you eat of whether or not your body really wants this food – that's the "how." Once that step is taken, then the "what" just follows along behind it like a shadow. Don't try to do everything at once, just pay attention to each food as it arises in your normal routine. By the end of the week, you'll be able to go back to your list of three columns and make some adjustments in the categories. That doesn't mean you have to throw out all the items in the "mind" column, although you might not reach for them so "mindlessly" the next time you pass them on the supermarket shelves. After all, you have the tools now to make changes and adjustments to your eating habits by following your own BodyWisdom, which knows much better than the latest diet book – or the current advertising campaign – about what is really right for you.

To help and inspire you to become more rooted in the "how" of eating – and in many of the other everyday activities we've talked about in this section – here are a couple of selections from Osho's talks on the subject.

"THE BODY CAN act totally; the mind can never act totally. Mind is always divided, mind works in dichotomies. So one part of the mind is angry, another part is simultaneously repenting or preparing to repent. This should also be noted – whenever there is a part constantly against another part, know that you are acting through the mind not through the body.

The body is total

Begin to do things bodily. When you are eating, eat bodily. The body knows well when to stop, but the mind never knows. One part will go on eating and another part will go on condemning. One part will go on saying stop, and another part will go on eating. The body is total, so ask the body. Do not ask the mind whether to eat or not to eat, to stop or not to stop. Your body knows what is needed. It has accumulated the wisdom of centuries and centuries. It knows when to stop.

Do not ask the mind, ask the body. Rely on the body's wisdom. The body is more wise than you. That is why animals live more wisely than us. They live more wisely, but, of course, they do not think. The moment they think they will be just like us. This is a miracle: that animals can live more wisely than human beings. It seems absurd. They know nothing, but they go on living more wisely. The only ability in which the human being has become efficient is to interfere with everything. You go on interfering with your body. Do not interfere, let the body work."[27]

Make contact with it

"You are not in contact with many things in your body, you are just carrying your body. Contact means a deep sensitivity. You may not even feel your body. It happens that only when you are ill do you feel your body. There is a headache, then you feel the head; without the headache there is no contact with the head. There is pain in the leg, you become aware of the leg. You become aware only when something goes wrong.

If everything is okay you remain completely unaware, and really, that is the moment when contact can be made – when everything is okay – because when something goes wrong then that contact is made with illness, with something that has gone wrong and the wellbeing is no more there. You have the head right now, then the headache comes and you make the contact. The contact is made not with the head but with the headache. With the head, contact is possible only when there is no headache and the head is filled with a wellbeing. But we have almost lost the capacity. We don't have any contact when we are okay. So our contact is just an emergency measure. There is a headache: some repair is needed, some medicine is needed, something has to be done, so you make the contact and do something.

Try to make contact with your body when everything is good. Just lie down on the grass, close the eyes, and feel the sensation that is going on within, the wellbeing that is bubbling. Lie down in a river. The water is touching the body and every cell is being cooled. Feel inside how that coolness enters cell by cell, goes deep into the body. The body is a great phenomenon, one of the miracles of nature.

Sit in the sun. Let the sunrays penetrate the body. Feel the warmth as it moves within, as it goes deeper, as it touches your blood cells and reaches to the very bones. And sun is life, the very source. So with closed eyes just feel what is happening. Remain alert, watch and enjoy. By and by you will become aware of a very subtle harmony, a very beautiful music continuously going on inside. Then you have the contact with the body; otherwise you carry a dead body. [28] "

The Couch Potato's Guide to Bodymind Fitness

MEDITATION BRINGS RELAXATION to the body and the mind. And, as we've mentioned before, the essence of meditation lies in watching – watching the movements of the body, the thoughts, the feelings. Just as though we were watching a film, or watching television. With an important difference, mind you – often, when we're watching a film or watching television we forget that we're watching. In fact, the most effective films draw us right into the action, make us laugh and cry, get excited or afraid. And as any woman knows – assuming she's not an avid football fan herself – even sports events on television can provoke the most ridiculous living-room behavior. Grown men have been observed to jump up and down, yell at referees and players who are hundreds of miles away, or even throw cans at the television screen.

We'll suggest a few things later on that you can do to give yourself little treats as you catch up with who's doing what to whom in your favorite soap opera. Just to get you started, though, is a simple exercise in reminding yourself that you're "watching." You might not want to use it all the time – that's half the fun, isn't it? getting so involved that you can forget yourself completely. But with scary, horrible, violent, tension-producing things like the evening news, this exercise comes in quite handy, and it's as simple as blinking your eyes.

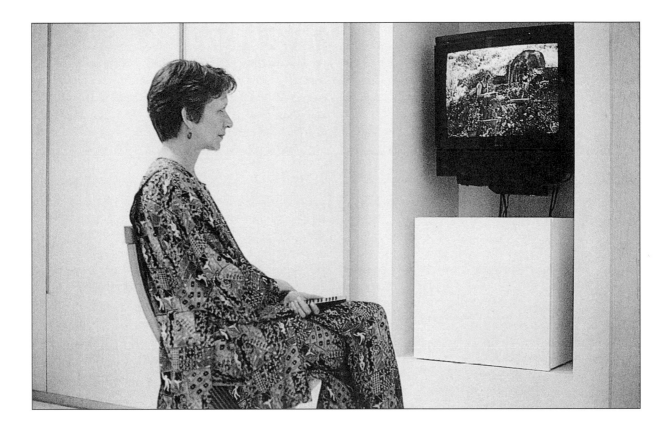

Just remind yourself, whenever you see something on the television or in a film that is a disturbance, to blink. Do it consciously, deliberately. Blink several times, and mentally remind yourself that it's a film. If it's real, like the evening news, remind yourself that it's not helpful for you to absorb this horror into your mind and body. It doesn't benefit either you or the situation being portrayed. Blink, and blink consciously. Experiment with doing it slowly, or more quickly, to see which works best for you. This isn't a showdown in the middle of the town square in an old Western movie – blink!

Come to think of it, if you discover that it works for you with the television, you might try it in life! Can't believe what's going on right before your very eyes? Blink!

Now, you've had enough TV but don't know what else to do? Here's something you can do without going any farther than the distance between the couch and the floor. It's an ancient Eastern technique, and Osho explains how it's done:

" This technique has been used by Taoists in China for centuries, and it is a wonderful technique – one of the easiest. Try this: *Without support for feet or hands, sit only on buttocks. Suddenly, the centring.*

What is to be done? You will need two things: first, a very sensitive body, which you do not have. You have a dead body; it is just a burden to be carried – not sensitive. First you will have to make your body sensitive; otherwise this technique will not work. So I will tell you something about how to make your body sensitive, and particularly your buttocks, because ordinarily your buttocks are the most insensitive part in your body. They have to be. They have to be because you are sitting the whole day on your buttocks. If they are too sensitive, it will be difficult.

So your buttocks are insensitive – they need to be. Just like the soles of the feet, they are insensitive. Continuously sitting on them, you never feel you are sitting on your buttocks. Have you ever felt it before this? Now you can feel you are sitting on your buttocks, but you have never felt it before – and you have been sitting on your buttocks your whole life, never aware. Their function is such that they cannot be very sensitive.

So first you have to make them sensitive. Try one very easy method... And this method can be done to any part of the body; then the body will become sensitive. Just sit on a chair, relaxed, and close your eyes. Feel your left hand or your right hand – either one. Feel your left hand. Forget the whole body and just feel the left hand. The more you feel it, the more the left hand will become heavy.

Go on feeling the left hand. Forget the whole body, just go on feeling the left hand as if you are just the left hand. The hand will go on becoming more and more and more heavy. As it goes on becoming heavy, go on feeling it becoming more heavy. Then try to feel what is happening in the hand. Whatever the sensation, note it down: any sensation, any jerk, any slight movement – note down in the mind that this is happening. And go on doing it every day for at least three weeks. At any time during the day, do it for ten minutes, 15 minutes. Just feel the left hand and forget the whole body.

Within three weeks you will feel you have a new left hand, or a new right hand. It will be so sensitive. And you will become aware of very minute and delicate sensations in the hand.

When you succeed with the hand, then try with the buttocks. Then try: close your eyes and feel that only two buttocks exist; you are no more. Let your whole consciousness go to the buttocks. It is not difficult. If you try, it is wonderful. And the feeling of aliveness that comes in the body is in itself very blissful. Then, when you can feel your buttocks and they can become very sensitive, when you can feel anything happening inside – a slight movement, a slight pain or anything – then you can observe and you can know. Then your consciousness is joined to the buttocks. First try it with the hand. Because the hand is very sensitive, it is easy. Once you gain the confidence that you can sensitize your hand, this confidence will help you to sensitize your buttocks. Then do this technique. So you will need at least six weeks before you can enter this technique – three weeks with your hand and then three weeks with your buttocks, just making them more and more sensitive.

Lying on the bed, forget the whole body. Just remember that only two buttocks are left. Feel the touch – the bedsheet, the coldness or the slowly coming warmth. Feel it. Lying down in your bathtub, forget the body. Remember only the buttocks – feel. Stand against a wall with your buttocks touching the wall – feel the coldness of the wall. Stand with your beloved, with your wife or husband, buttock to buttock – feel the other through the buttocks. This is just to "create" your buttocks, to bring them to a situation where they start feeling.

Then do this technique: *Without support for feet or hands... Sit on the ground. Without support for feet or hands, sit only on the buttocks.* The Buddha posture will do... any ordinary posture will do, but it is good not to use your hands. Just remain on the buttocks; sit only on the buttocks. Then what to do? Just close your eyes. Feel the buttocks touching the ground. And because the buttocks have become sensitive, you will feel that one buttock is touching more. You are leaning on one buttock, and the other is touching less. Then move the leaning to the other. Immediately move to the other; then come to the first. Go on moving from one to the other, and then by and by, balance.

Balancing means that both of your buttocks are feeling the same. Your weight on both of the buttocks is exactly the same. And when your buttocks are sensitive this will not be difficult, you will feel it. Once both your buttocks are balanced, *suddenly, the centring.* With that balance, suddenly you will be thrown to your navel centre, and you will be centred inside. You will forget the buttocks, you will forget the body. You will be thrown to the inner centre....

You have seen buddhas sitting. You may not have imagined that they are balancing their buttocks. You go to a temple and see Mahavir sitting, Buddha sitting; you may never have imagined that this sitting is just a balancing on the buttocks. It is – and when there is no imbalance, suddenly that balance gives you the centring. [29] ”

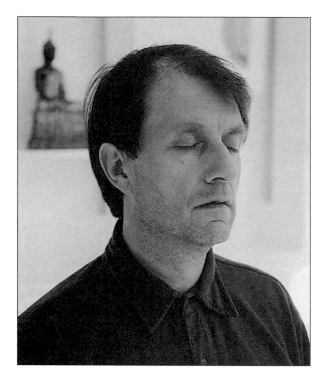

ONE OF THE most common excuses we use for not taking better care of ourselves is that we "don't have time." And one of the things that takes up plenty of our time at home is sitting in front of the television! Right, we know that it's sometimes even educational. It's also a great opportunity give yourself a few small treats that don't even require you to get up off the couch.

1 This is good to do during station breaks and commercials, because you can close your eyes. It needs a good imagination, and may be difficult for some people. But give it a try, and if you can get the knack it's a tremendous relaxation for the eyes. Close your eyes, and imagine that strings are attached to the back of your eyeballs. From there, they pass through little pulleys at the back of your skull, where they hang down because there are small weights attached to the ends of the string. Let the weights just pull gently on the back of the eyeballs, and feel how it relaxes the eyes and pulls your attention right inside. Be careful... you might enjoy it so much that you miss the rest of the programme!

2 It's certainly more fun to have somebody else massage your head, but it's quite simple to do yourself, and you can feel what's happening from the inside and adjust accordingly. The secret to a really refreshing and relaxing head massage is to move the skin separately from the skull. On most people, because there's so much tension stored in the head, this is not easy to do. We're so busy trying to keep our heads together that the scalp seems to be glued to the skull.

It's not, really, though. And if you work on it from time to time, it will loosen up by and by, with a corresponding relaxation that spreads all through the body. Try it with your own head – does the scalp move easily? Forward and backward, from side to side? Use firm pressure with all the five fingers of both hands, not "rubbing" the scalp but actually trying to shift it. Don't be discouraged if it doesn't move much – just persuade it a little, slowly and sensitively. Do it whenever you think of it, and be sure not to tense your arms and shoulders in the process. Try it in front of the mirror, too, if that helps you get the hang of it.

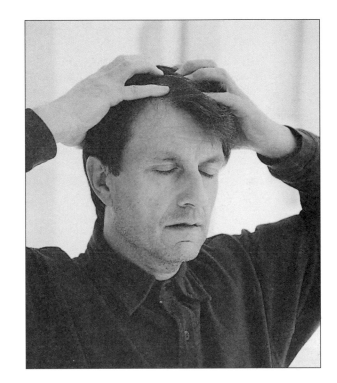

HERE IS AN exercise you can do to explore a new and unfamiliar dimension of watching, looking. It comes from the Secret of the Golden Flower, an ancient Taoist book of mysteries, and detailed instructions for the exercise are given by Osho.

Master Lu-tsu said:
When the light is made to move in a circle, all the energies of heaven and earth, of the light and the dark, are crystallized.

"YOUR CONSCIOUSNESS IS flowing outward — this is a fact, there is nothing to believe or disbelieve about it. When you look at an object, your consciousness flows towards the object. For example, you are looking at me — then you forget yourself, you become focused on me. Then your energy flows towards me, then your eyes are arrowed towards me. This is extroversion. You see a flower and you are enchanted, and you become focused on the flower. You become oblivious of yourself, you are only attentive to the beauty of the flower.

This we know — every moment it is happening. A beautiful woman passes by and suddenly your energy starts following her. We know this outward flow of light, but this is only half of the story. Each time the light flows out, you fall into the background, you become oblivious of yourself.

The light has to flow back so that you are both the subject and the object at the same time, simultaneously, so that you see yourself. Then self-knowledge is released. Ordinarily, we live only in this half way — half-alive, half-dead, that's the situation. Slowly slowly, light goes on flowing outward and never returns. You become more and more empty inside, hollow. You become a black hole.

This is exactly what happens on a greater scale in the universe. Physicists have now discovered black holes. Taoists discovered black holes long before, but they were not concerned about the black holes there in the faraway space, they were concerned about the black holes inside you. A black hole is a state when all your energy is spent, exhausted, and you have become empty and you have forgotten completely how to go on nourishing this source of energy. Scientists say that sooner or later our sun will become a black hole, because energy is continuously being released but nothing is returning to it. It is an immense source of energy — for millions of years it has been giving light to the solar system. For millions of years trees have been growing, flowers flowering, man living, animals moving, birds flying, because of the sun's energy. But the sun is becoming spent. One day it will collapse; there will be no more energy left. Suddenly all light will disappear, the last rays will disappear from it. Then it will be a black hole.

And that's how many people live their life: they become black holes because of this constant extroversion. You see this, you see that, you are continuously seeing without ever returning the energy to the seer. In the day you see the world, in the night you see dreams, but you go on remaining constantly attached to objects. This is dissipating energy....

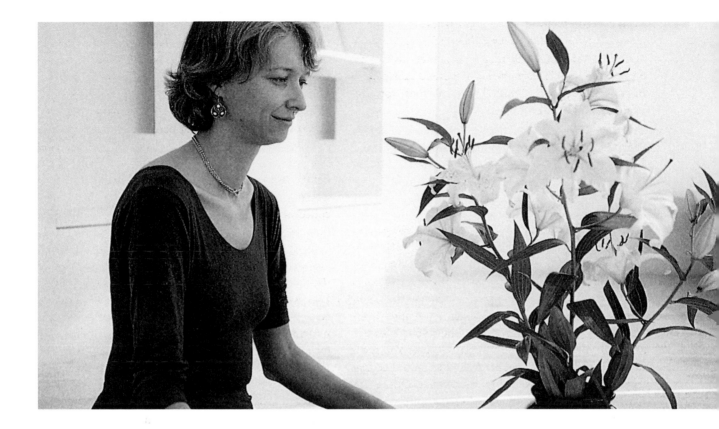

The Taoist experience is that this energy that you spend in your extroversion can be more and more crystallized, rather than spent, if you learn the secret science of turning it backwards. It is possible; that is the whole science of all methods of concentration.

Just standing before a mirror some day, try one small experiment. You are looking at the mirror, your own face in the mirror, your own eyes in the mirror. This is extroversion: you are looking into the mirrored face — your own face but it is an object outside you. Then, for a moment, reverse the whole process. Start feeling that you are being looked at by the reflection in the mirror — not that you are looking at the reflection but the reflection is looking at you — and you will be in a very strange space.

Just try it for a few minutes and you will be very alive, and something of immense power will start entering you. You may even become frightened because you have never known it; you have never seen the complete circle of energy.

Although it is not mentioned in Taoist scriptures this seems to me the most simple experiment anybody can do, and very easily. Just standing before the mirror in your bathroom, first look into the reflection: you are looking and the reflection is the object. Then change the whole situation, reverse the process. Start feeling that you are the reflection and the reflection is looking at you, and immediately you will see a change happening, a great energy moving towards you.

In the beginning it may be frightening because you have never done it and you have never known it; it will look crazy. You may feel shaken, a trembling may arise in you, or you may feel disorientated, because your whole orientation up to now has been extroversion. Introversion has to be learned slowly. But the circle is complete, and if you do it for a few days you will be surprised how much more alive you feel the whole day. Just a few minutes standing before the mirror and letting the energy come back to you so the circle is complete...

Whenever the circle is complete there is a great silence. The incomplete circle creates restlessness. When the circle is complete it creates rest, it makes you centered. And to be centered is to be powerful – the power is yours. This is just an experiment; then you can try it in many ways.

Looking at the rose flower, first look at the rose flower for a few moments, a few minutes, and then start the reverse process: the rose flower is looking at you. You will be surprised how much energy the rose flower can give to you. And the same can be done with trees and the stars and with people. The best way is to do it with the woman or man you love. Just look into each other's eyes. First begin looking at the other and then start feeling the other returning the energy to you; the gift is coming back. You will feel replenished, you will feel showered, bathed, basked in a new kind of energy. You will come out of it rejuvenated, vitalized.[30]

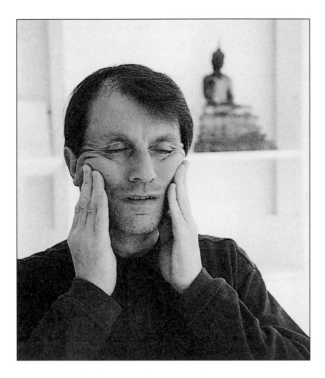 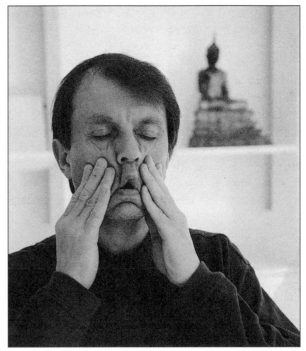

Take Off a Happy Face

YOU'VE JUST GOT home from the party. You've been smiling so much – that particular kind of smile that's just on the lips and not from the heart – that your face aches. Or, you've spent the whole day driving around in traffic that would cause even a saint to behave like Attilla the Hun, and you feel like your jaw has been wired together. It's time to take off your face and relax! The secret to a really relaxing face massage – and one that doesn't give you even more wrinkles than you've just earned in that traffic jam – is to remember to go for the muscles, not the skin. Plant your fingers gently but deeply into the muscles and just move them around – up, down, in little circles. Work slowly and thoroughly, across every inch of the face, reaching in for the muscles and gently helping each to relax. Yes, you can do this in front of the television – but it might be more enjoy able with your eyes closed, giving it your total attention.

"Take work as a game and enjoy it. Everything is a challenge. Just don't go on doing it, dragging yourself because it has to be done. Then you will become ill. If you have to work for four, five hours a day and those hours are a continuous sub current of avoiding it, then you are dividing your being. It is not a question of work. It is a question of your whole inner well-being. You will become divided doing something for four or five hours which you cannot like or don't like.

So there are only two possibilities: either find work you like or become capable of liking the work, whatsoever it is. The second is the best alternative because it is very difficult to find work that you like. Sooner or later you will dislike it...because every kind of work, by and by becomes boring, you have to repeat everything. The other alternative is best. Bring a capability to like anything that you do; whatsoever the work you can like it.

Try it. Find ways to like it. People want to find ways to dislike it, so of course they find ways. For three weeks, try doing the work and liking it. Enjoy it, and singingly. Let it be just a dance. If you are cleaning, it can be a dance, a singing, an enjoyment, a delight and you will be tremendously benefited by it."[31]

The Handyman's Drill

IF YOU SPEND your weekends tinkering with engines, doing carpentry or cabinet-work, mowing the lawn, or polishing the car, you can develop a few kinks from using the body in ways that are uncommon to your everyday routine. We offer two quick fixes in this section for common afflictions of the "man around the house."

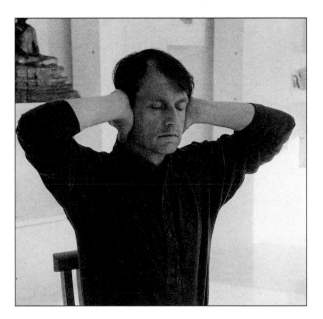

1 This is a repeat from the office section, just in case you passed it by because it didn't seem to apply to you. It's great for giving the hands and wrists a treat when you've spent the past hour fiddling in impossibly small places. The effect is to open the energy flow through the wrists. Grasp the back of one hand with the opposite hand as shown, and pull gently around in a circular motion. To give a little added stretch, pull both hands down towards your waist. This is actually

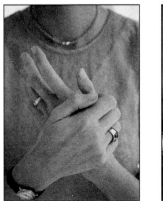
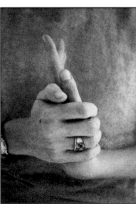

a martial arts exercise, and helps to bring the energy to the "hara" center just below the navel.

2 If your ears are ringing from the sound of the circular saw, the drill or the lawnmower, try this to restore a bit of peace and quiet to your frazzled senses. Just cover both ears with the palms of your hands and press firmly, so that you shut out all noises from the outside. Now quickly remove the hands from your ears – voilà! You've got your hearing back, and as an added bonus, the static and tension in your brain can start to dissolve, too.

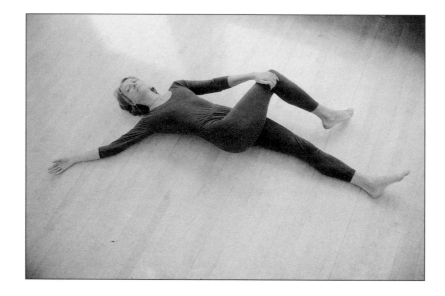

3 When you've been standing or sitting for a long time, especially if you've been concentrating on a task and not noticing that you've become tense in the legs or lower back, you can develop a pain that seems to run from the lower back or buttocks all the way down the back of one leg. That's a sign that your sciatic nerve is being pinched. In some people it can become a chronic and very painful condition. But often it's a fairly simple thing to fix, with the stretching exercise pictured opposite.

Lie down on the floor or on a very firm mattress, and just settle in and let yourself relax for a few moments, observing the breath and consciously letting go of any tensions you can feel in the body. When you're ready, raise one leg and wrap your arms around the knees as shown, pulling the leg firmly towards your chest until you feel a pleasant stretch from your lower back down through the leg. Notice the angle of the leg in the photo opposite – this is

important, because it is at this angle, or the angle very near it that is perfect for you, that the pressure on the sciatic nerve is easily released. Go slowly, be sensitive to how your body is feeling, and don't force anything beyond that point of pleasurable pain. Once you've tried it a few times, you'll know exactly how to do it – but you should always take it easy, or you run the risk of making things even worse. When you've found just the right spot – if you stay in contact with your body, it will tell you – hold the leg there, and breathe deeply a few times. Feel the slight increase in the stretch as you breathe in, and consciously relax the lower back and the buttocks as you breathe out. Now release the leg slowly, and return it gently to the floor. Rest there a few moments, and then repeat the whole process with the other leg. When you've done both legs, you can rest for as long as you like with your feet flat on the floor, and your knees up. To get up, roll over on your side first and come up slowly.

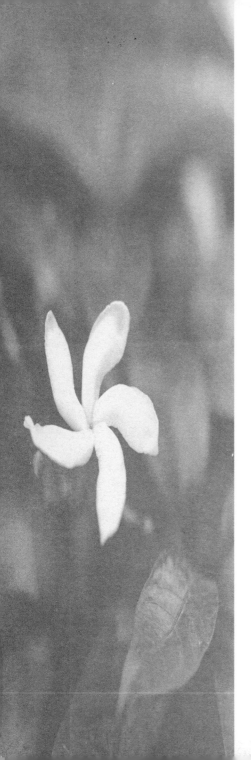

"Fishes are not as foolish as man. They simply live, they enjoy, they eat, drink and are merry. They dance. They are so grateful for the littlest pond that has been given to them. They delight in it. Look at the fishes in a pond. Jumping, delighting, running hither and thither. It seems there is no goal for them, no ambition, their needs are fulfilled. When they are tired, they move into the shadow in pond and pool. They rest. When energy comes they move and dance and float and swim; when they are tired again, they move into the shadow and rest. Their life is a rhythm between rest and action.

You have lost the rhythm. You act but there is no rest. You go to the shop but you never come back home — even if you come, the shop comes in your head. You never seek a shadow in the pond, in the pool. That is all that meditation is — to seek the pond, the shadow."[32]

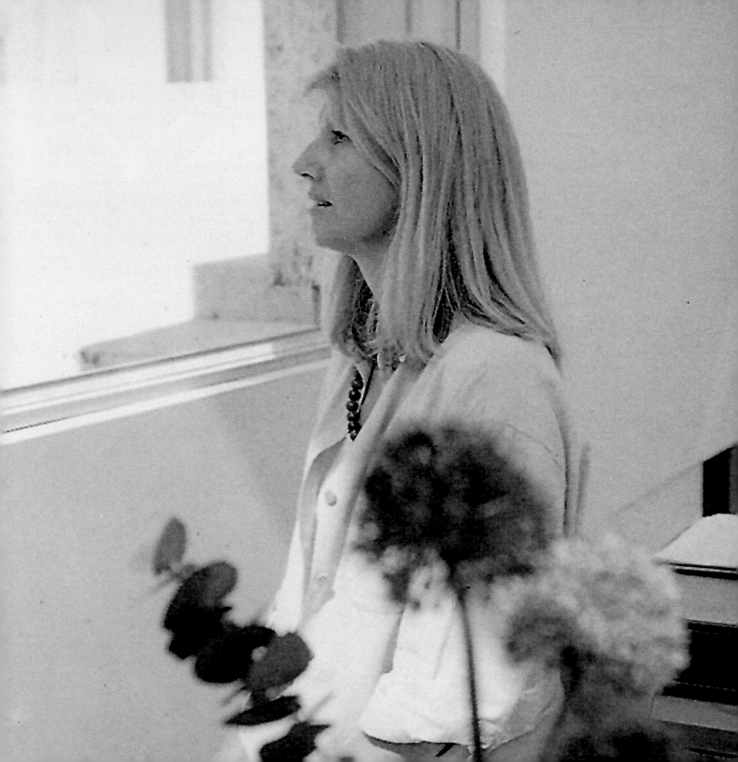

Home Spa Recipes for the Tense and the Tired

EVERY EVENING WHEN we come home, we have a choice: we can either continue to carry the day in our heads, or we can leave it outside the door. We can either slip out of our work and get into something more comfortable, or we can spend the whole evening in the neckties and nylons of our mental list of "to-dos."

It's not always easy to choose the more relaxed option. And sometimes we really do have to quite literally bring our work home in order to finish the tasks of the day. But believe it or not, it doesn't add a thing to anybody's mental effectiveness to be running the mind full throttle 18 hours a day. It gets tired, and when it gets tired it doesn't function so well. We know that, actually. That's why we so often throw ourselves down in front of the television, or turn on the radio, or try to create any kind of distraction in the hope that we can derail the mind from its tracks for at least a few moments and give it a break.

The weekends are a good time to try an alternative experiment: Just allow yourself a day to do exactly what you feel like doing, in whatever order it comes up, putting aside everything else on your list. If you feel like starting that book, do it. If you feel like lying around on the couch all day, why not? If it's a nice day, why not go out somewhere and find a patch of grass where you can lie on your back and watch the clouds? You might even find yourself overcome by an urge to deep clean the garage — that's great,

too! You don't have to spend your day in "pointless" activities, it's just that you will allow whatever urge arises from someplace other than your mind. See if you can discover your own rhythms of action and rest, rest and action, by putting aside all your habitual routines and allowing something completely new to emerge.

It's a bit like the "Moving From Within" exercise earlier in the book, only expanded and enlarged to encompass all the activities of your day. Just tell yourself you're going to wake up in the morning with no plans, no ideas about what to do or where to go, and see where your day takes you when you let yourself be taken. Go into it with a real openness and innocence. If you can manage to persuade your mind to leave you alone — you can make a promise to the mind: "It's just for this one day" — you'll probably make quite a few discoveries about what you really like to do and not-do.

"RELAXATION MEANS YOU don't have any shoulds. You are simply living moment to moment, not according to some future idea of yourself, but according to your reality that is herenow. To live with the reality, moment to moment, is to be sane. To live with the idea is to be insane....

The goal-oriented idea is driving you mad. Drop that idea, and suddenly you will see sanity explodes into your being.

You start laughing again. You start dancing again…

We are not going anywhere! We are here! And we have been here for the whole of eternity and we are going to be here for the whole of eternity. Now it is up to you to enjoy or not to enjoy. We are here and we are going to be here. There is no way to escape. Now it is for you to choose whether to enjoy or just to cry and weep for the goal.

The goal is not; there is no goal…. If the world had any goal, it would have achieved it by now. How long it has existed! The very fact that it has not achieved it yet is proof enough that it has no goal to achieve. It simply goes on; it is an ongoing affair. It is not a film that comes to an end, it is not a novel that comes to an end. We are always in the middle, never in the beginning and never at the end. We are always in the middle. And that is the way things are.

So the goal-oriented person misses all that is beautiful in life. The goal he cannot achieve because there is no goal, and on the way he misses all things. Have you watched? Sometimes you are rushing towards the market, to your shop or to your office, you pass through the same street where you go for a morning walk, or sometimes in the moonlit night you go for a stroll – the same road, the same trees – but when you are going to the office you have a goal in mind; then you don't see the greenery and then you don't listen to the birds. You are not interested in the way; you are interested in the goal. You want to finish it any way. The faster you can go,

the better. You will not like to walk to the office. You go in a car or in a bus.

And if someday science manages to materialize and dematerialize man, you will simply stand in a machine in your house and dematerialize there and materialize in the office – so no need for the way. One day it is going to happen. There is no need to go. Immediately, from one place to another place you can have a quantum leap, a quantum jump. In the middle you will not be. Speed – because you are not interested in the way.

But, the same way, in the morning when you go for a walk, has a totally different quality. You enjoy it. Each breeze passing through the trees and each bird flying around. You enjoy it because you are not going anywhere in particular. You are just going for a morning walk. It is playful. You can turn back from any point. There is no goal in your mind. You are non-tense, you are relaxed. There is joy, there is poetry. You start singing a song.

You can treat yourself on the way of life in these two ways. If you are goal oriented – God, heaven, moksha, nirvana, whatsoever you call it – then you cannot enjoy, you cannot celebrate on the way. Zen says the way is the goal. That is the meaning when they say the samsara is nirvana. The way is the goal, so don't miss anything. Enjoy. Each moment has to be tasted; each moment is delicious. Each moment brings something to you, a blessing, a benediction. Don't miss it.[33]

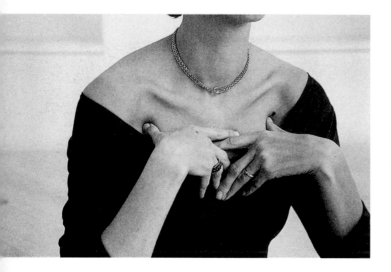

THESE SPOTS ON the chest are known as "let-go points" – and that's just what they help you to do. When you find yourself "holding on" to something – whether it is something unpleasant that happened during the day, or an unhappy memory that just won't seem to go away – these points can help you to relax your hold and let go. These let-go points on the chest help to release both physical and psychological tensions that are no longer useful to us in dealing with a painful experience. We all get hurt, we all feel sad sometimes. Many more problems arise from repressing and judging these emotions than from the emotions themselves. If we can "let go" of them in a safe and comfortable environment, they will soon pass away.

The points are located roughly at the place shown by our model in the photograph on this page, on the upper – outside portion of your chest. Explore around a bit until you find the knots there – these points usually are painful, because most of us are usually "holding on" to something or another! Apply enough pressure to feel a pleasurable pain, and hold the points for a few moments, breathing into them to increase the pressure and letting go of more and more tension and pain with each out breath. It's also fine to massage the points, and it is a nice thing to do with a trusted friend.

THIS IS A wonderfully womb-like posture, very restful and somehow reassuring. Notice that the legs are folded, and the arms are lying loose at the sides.

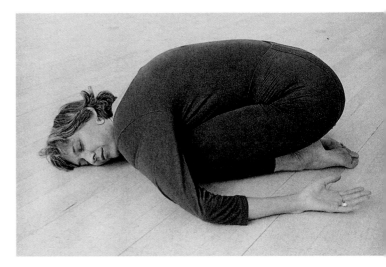

In this posture, you'll find that you become easily aware of where in your body you are still holding tension   and the posture is one that helps you to easily relax the tension being held and let it go. It's particularly good for opening and relaxing the neck, spine and lower back – and it also helps your breathing to become deeper and more natural, as your lungs expand and contract against the pressure of your thighs on the chest.

Be aware to keep your knees together in this posture, and to relax the ankles so the heels fall apart naturally. Let the buttocks sink back onto the heels, or if this is not possible, feel that the buttocks are sinking towards the earth.

If you are carrying a lot of tension in the neck and you experience uncomfortable pain, you can try putting a small pillow between the legs and the chest. This should lessen the amount of stretch in the neck and help you to feel more comfortable. Turn the head from one side to the other, so that both sides of the neck and shoulders are stretched. Feel free to rest in the posture as long as you like.

Some people find this a nice posture to move into on waking up in the morning, too – especially those mornings when you're reluctant to get up! It's just the right sort of reassurance and support to help you face the day...

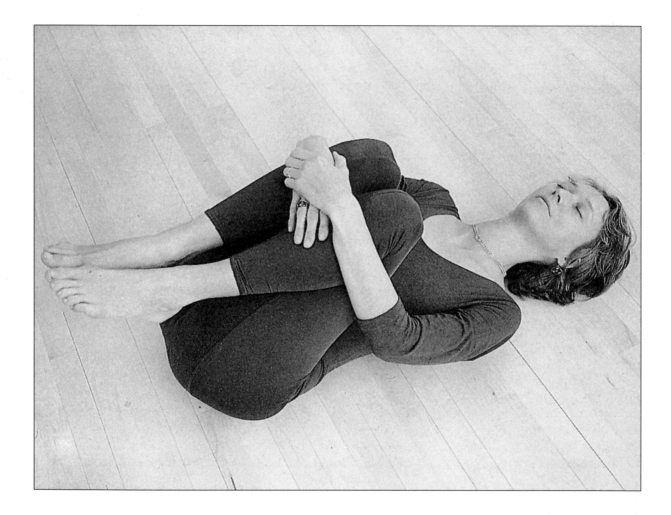

The posture pictured opposite is a real treat for those of us who suffer from lower back pain, and it is almost as womb-like and reassuring as the posture pictured on the previous page. Just lie on your back — best without a pillow, though you could roll up a towel to fit under your neck if you feel too uncomfortable without any support there — and raise your knees, wrapping your arms comfortably around the knees. Let the weight of your arms pull the knees towards your chest, "breathing into" the spine and lower back. This posture can also help to release tension from the upper back and shoulders, so check to make sure that you are using the arms and not using the shoulders to hold the knees to your chest.

"THOSE WHO HAVE again arrived to the same state of silence, peace and tranquility as a child in the mother's womb — in other words, the people for whom the whole existence has become a womb, a mother — all these people have found it to be as if they have come back home: a vaster home, with more freedom, with immense space, with great beauty, with intense ecstasy.

The old home was just a far-away echo of the real home. The real home is to find one's solitude, to find one's aloneness, to find oneself.

We are wandering always outside, going somewhere. And every going is going away from yourself. You may be going in search of a home, but in fact you are going away from home — your home is within you. And that home can be found only when you stop searching, when you stop wandering, when you are no longer interested in the distant but utterly relaxed in your very source of being.

The home is to be found within you. And solitude is an essential, a basic necessity. To be with yourself — that's what is the meaning of solitude. We know how to be with others, we know how to be in a crowd, but we have forgotten the language of being with oneself.

This is not loneliness, because loneliness is always asking for the other. Loneliness is painful. Loneliness is not a rest, but a restlessness. Loneliness is not the home; the home is aloneness.[34]"

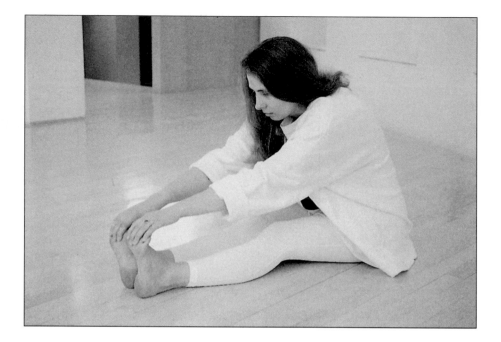

THE MERIDIANS IN the body are, according to oriental medicine, the pathways taken by the "chi" or vital energy. The meridians are used in acupuncture and shiatsu to locate places where the flow of chi might be blocked. A blockage usually corresponds to a difficulty in one or more of the organs of the body. When we experience discomfort or illness, the flow of energy through the meridians can be checked to determine which of the organs are likely to be in distress.

The "meridian stretches" in this section of *BodyWisdom* will help to open up and strengthen the blockages in energy flow caused by tension, improper diet or illness. Listen to your body when you try them – it knows what feels good, and what feels good is almost certainly what it needs. The only specific caution is not to "bounce" in any of the positions. Just take the stretch as far as you can, to the point where you feel a pleasurable sort of pain.

1 The kidney/bladder meridian stretch will feel good to almost everybody, since when we get exhausted and depleted the kidneys and bladder are usually the first organs to suffer. This stretch is done by putting your legs straight out in front of you, and touching your toes with your hands. Next, the idea is to bend forward and touch your head to your knees!

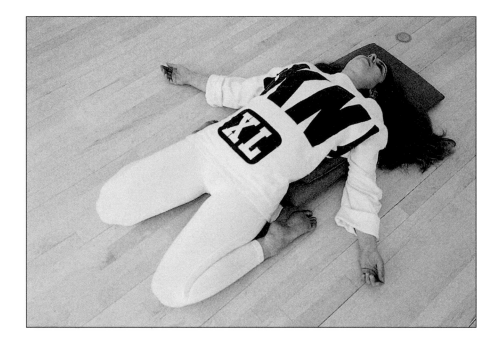

Don't worry if you can't do it at first – just go as far as you can, and when you've reached that point allow yourself to relax into the stretch and take a couple of deep breaths, letting the relaxation deepen with each outbreath. Come back up slowly, and try again tomorrow. Day by day, you'll find that you're able to go forward just a little more – but the real point is the stretch, so don't worry about your progress, just enjoy!

2 Here, we've pictured the easy bit of the stomach/spleen meridian stretch, which is the lying down part. If you've got good stomach muscles and a strong back, you can start this stretch by sitting on your knees Japanese-style, raising your clasped hands high over your head and, keeping the back straight, going backwards till your back lies flat on the floor. Try it, and if it's impossible, then it's fine just to manoeuvre yourself into the position as best you can, taking care not to strain the lower back. Once you're there, take a couple of deep breaths and feel the stretching all down the front of the torso and thighs.

The stomach/spleen meridian is connected with our "doing" – when it's out of balance we can go into workaholic hyperspeed, or we can feel so exhausted that all we want to do is lie down.

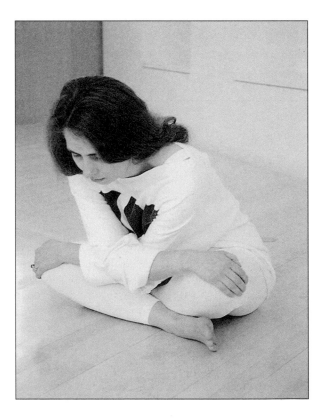

3 The heart constrictor/triple heater meridian stretch is a great tonic for the whole body, improving circulation and our ability to make the best use of the nutrients we take in. Sit with your legs crossed, and the hands placed on the opposite knees. Bend forward as far as possible – the idea is that your head should touch the floor, but it might take a while before you can reach that point. Just let the weight of your head stretch you out as far as you can go, and then breathe deeply a couple of times, relaxing more into the stretch with each out breath.

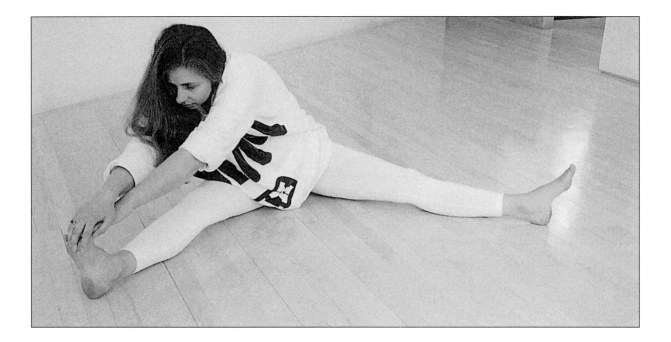

4 This exercise stretches the liver and gall bladder meridians. When we have trouble concentrating – or tend to get upset when our concentration is disturbed – it's often because the energy flowing through these meridians is disturbed or blocked in some way. The stretch helps to balance things out, and also enhances the body's ability to deal with the toxins we're exposed to through our food or the environment. Sitting on the floor, spread your legs as far apart as they will go. Now reach out to touch your toes, going as far as you can without bending the knees. Once you get to the maximum stretch point, relax into it and take a couple of deep breaths, allowing yourself to sink a little more deeply into the stretch as you breathe out. Now repeat the movement in the direction of the other leg.

5 The "kidney flush" which helps the kidney to release accumulated toxins and function more efficiently. As you breathe in, imagine that your breath is going to the kidneys and circulating through them. Hold yourself in the posture by keeping the spine straight, while at the same time imagining that you are pushing yourself forward from the kidneys toward the front of the body. It's rather like imagining the kidneys are a sponge, and you're squeezing them out. It's important to keep the spine straight, and to hold this position for not longer than one minute.

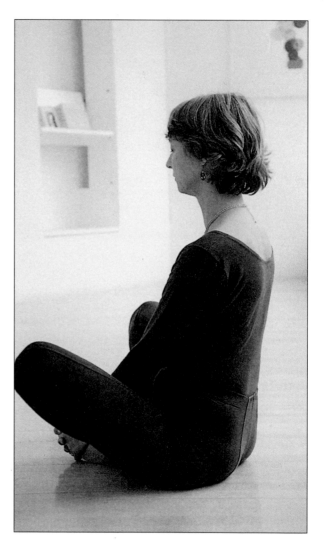

THE HEALTHY FUNCTIONING of the kidneys makes a tremendous difference to how we feel. Whenever you feel tired or lethargic during the day, reach first for a glass of water – not ordinary tap water, but filtered or spring water, please! – and drink it. Chances are most of your tiredness and lethargy will have vanished within fifteen minutes or so. In oriental systems of medicine, the kidneys are the "reservoir of chi" – the pool of energy that feeds all the other energy systems in the body. In the posture pictured here, keep your spine straight, and pull your heels as close to your body as possible. This will help direct the energy of the breath towards the kidneys, so the exercise can work as it is intended to.

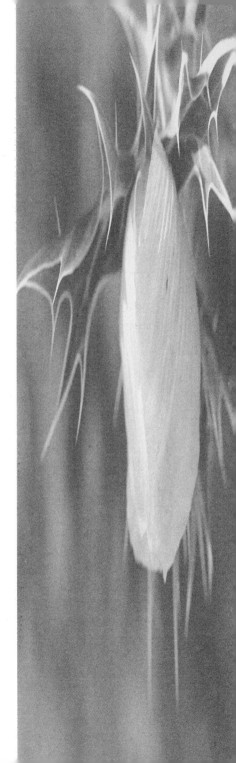

"Man is in the body but is not the body. The body is beautiful, the body has to be loved and respected, but one has not to forget that one is not it, that one is just a resident in the body. The body is a temple: it is a host to you, but you are not part of it. The body is a contribution from the earth; you come from the sky. In you, as in every embodied being, the earth and the sky are meeting: it is a love affair of earth and sky." [35]

Sleepy Body, Sweet Dreams

"THERE ARE CERTAIN things which, if you try to do, you will undo. If you don't try to do them you may be able to do them. The very effort leads you to the reverse effect. For example, sleep. You want to go to sleep – what can you do? Everybody has a fundamental right to sleep, but what can you do? Can you ask the police to come and help? What can you do when you don't feel like going to sleep? Whatsoever you do is going to disturb you because the very effort works against sleep. Sleep is an effortlessness. When you simply relax, not doing anything, by and by you drift into sleep. You cannot swim towards it – you drift. You cannot make any conscious effort.

And this is the problem with all those people who suffer from sleeplessness, insomnia. All insomniacs have their rituals. They do certain things to cause sleep to come to them. And that is where they miss, that is where everything goes wrong. How can you force sleep? The more you force the more you will be there – aware, alert, conscious. Every effort will make you more aware, more alert, and sleep will be put off. What do you do when you want to go to sleep? You don't do anything. You simply wait, in a restful mood. You simply allow sleep to come to you – you cannot force it. You cannot demand, you cannot say, "Come!" With closed eyes, in a dark room, on your pillow, you simply wait... and waiting, you start drifting. Like a cloud glides, drifts, you drift by and by from the conscious mind to the unconscious.

You lose all control. You have to lose control; otherwise you cannot go to sleep, because the part that controls is the conscious mind. It has to allow. Control has to be left completely. Then – you don't know when and why and how – sleep comes to you. Only in the morning you become aware that you have been asleep, and you slept well.[36] "

SLEEPLESSNESS IS A peculiarly modern disease. In part it is because we don't use our bodies much, so we rarely experience the pleasant tiredness that comes from strenuous physical activity. The fact that our minds are so busy all day long doesn't help, either. It takes the mind a while to slow down, like a bicycle we've been pedalling very fast downhill. And if we can't find ways to allow the mind to slow down but rather try to stop it forcibly, to make it go to sleep, it will put up a fight!

So, we're not going to give you methods for falling asleep in this section of the book. Rather, we're going to show you some ways you can help the body and mind let go of their tensions so your sleep can bring you more rest and relaxation.

As you experiment with the techniques, don't think of them as ways to bring on sleep. As Osho points out at the beginning of this section, one of the most counter-productive things we can do when we have trouble sleeping is to make a problem out of it, and add the tension of "trying to get to sleep" to the other tensions we are already carrying.

When the body is too tense to let go into sleep, it lets us know by tossing and turning. We can't get comfortable, no matter which way we turn, and the arms and legs – so helpful and compliant in the daytime – suddenly seem to have developed a mind of their own. For this situation, the simple methods we've pictured on the following pages will be helpful.

For the racing-downhill mind, here are a few things to do. Remember, we're not saying that by doing them you'll be able to go to sleep! But they might help you to at least stop pedalling the bicycle, and at the very least they'll give you something else to do besides worry about the fact that it's bedtime and you have an important meeting in the morning, and you can't sleep.

1 The hands are very closely tied to the brain, and one way to help release the tensions of the brain is to release the tensions in the hands. After you get into bed, and before lying down on the pillow, take a few minutes just to let your hands play. Have fun with it – imagine you're playing the piano, make little shadow animals with them on the wall. Pretend you're a Balinese or Indian dancer, and tell stories with your hands. Just let the hands express whatever is inside, let them dance, let them fly.

2 If it's possible for you to do without disturbing the neighbors, and if you can give yourself the privacy and space to do it, gibberish is a great way to release the tensions of the mind. Just make nonsense sounds, blabla leedadida gfurzpltz gleeb... you get the idea. Let it start out softly, as though you're singing a little song to yourself, and then let yourself really get into it.

Absurd and silly, yes! – and let yourself laugh, use the energy of the laughter to go into it even more. Have all the nonsense conversations you like, and let your body move if it wants to move. Pound on the pillows, wave your arms around, become a raving maniac! Whew! That feels better, doesn't it?

And finally, here's a method given by Osho. It's good for those times when the day has been really full, and you can't quite seem to let it go.

" Every night before you go to sleep, finish that day. It is finished in existence; now it is futile to carry it in the mind. Just be finished with it. Say goodbye to it. If something has remained incomplete in the day it is difficult to finish it. Complete it, complete it in the mind. You were passing on the road and you saw a beautiful woman and you wanted to hug her. Now that cannot be done; something hangs incomplete.

Before you go to sleep just look at the whole day and see what is incomplete. Complete it psychologically: hug her. Relive that moment, hug her in the mind, thank her and be finished with it! Don't carry it incomplete. Only incomplete moments are carried. They hang, because each experience wants to be complete.

There is an intrinsic mechanism in each and everything that compels it to become complete. A seed wants to become the tree, a child wants to become a young man, the unripe fruit wants to become ripe, and so on and so forth. Everything wants to complete itself; it has a built-in urge to complete. And that is so about every experience.

You wanted to hit somebody and it was not feasible, not practical. It would have cost too much and you were not ready to lose that much. Do it before you go to sleep. Let there be 30 minutes every night, and that will be your meditation: go on finishing. Start from the morning and finish everything that has remained incomplete. You will be surprised that it can be completed. And once it has been completed you will fall into sleep. By and by you will see that dreams are disappearing, because dreams are a mechanism, a natural mechanism to complete things... but then things are completed very unconsciously.

In a very, very primitive way the dreams try to complete what you are not doing. Dreams are great helpers; they complement your existence in many ways. You wanted to hug the woman: you will hug the woman in the dream but it will be an unconscious thing. Maybe in the morning you will forget about it, you may not remember it. The mind that wanted to hug is the conscious mind and the mind that hugged is the unconscious. They may never meet; the message may never be delivered. There are a thousand and one barriers for the message to reach.

So in the unconscious it has been completed but in the conscious it remains incomplete. A hankering and a longing goes on and on. There are many things clamouring for your attention and this load becomes bigger and bigger every day and then it is almost impossible to finish it. From tonight start finishing things every day. And within two, three months your dreams will start completely disappearing. When dreams start disappearing that is an indication that meditation is working.

I am not interested in analysing dreams; I am interested in helping them to disappear. That's the difference between psychoanalysis and meditation, between the western psychology and the eastern psychology. For nearly three thousand years we have been working on how to help dreams to disappear. Once dreams are gone completely you have a clarity, your mind is unclouded, but the way to help the dreams go is to complete things consciously, otherwise they will be there.

If you have completed things there is no need for them to be there. Then the sleep becomes deep sleep – what in yoga is called *sushupti* – a dreamless sleep.[37] "

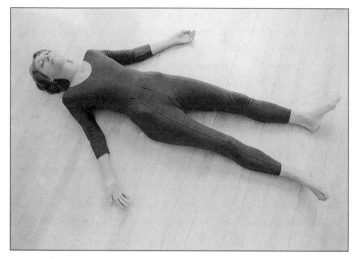

experiment you'll be developing this knack of watching, and the watchfulness will continue through the whole night. Then, when you wake up in the morning, you'll see: your mind tends to just pick up where it left off the night before. And you can see it, because the thread of watchfulness is in your hands.

That's how these relaxation techniques work with the body, in the same way. When you fall asleep with the body in a state of relaxation, the relaxation continues throughout the night. You're less likely to wake up in the morning feeling tired, or with a kink in your back or shoulder. So just experiment with them to see what works best for you... and choose the ones your body likes.

THE REST OF the exercises in this section are to help your body unwind the tensions of the day, so that you can relax. The easiest time to do them is just before you go to sleep – but really, they can be done any time when you're feeling particularly tense or "wound up."

Osho has pointed out – and you can try it as an experiment for yourself – that the last thought we have before actually slipping out of the conscious mind and down into sleep, is the first thought we'll have when we come out of sleep and back into the conscious mind in the morning.

We're not always aware of our thoughts, of course, so it might not be obvious that this is true. But if you can develop the knack of watching – not getting involved, not following the thoughts here and there, but just watching them – you'll see how they begin to slow down. If you enjoy the

PICTURED ON THIS PAGE:
This is a standard relaxation technique that works really well, because it engages the help of the mind in relaxing the body. Find a comfortable position on your back, with your arms to your sides.

Spend a few moments just letting your breathing settle into a natural, easy rhythm. Now look around for places in the body which are obviously holding some tension, and consciously let the tension go. You'll find that after you do this, you feel a bit more settled into the mattress, and the body feels a bit heavier.

Now go to the feet, and start from there on an inner journey through the body to explore where you still might be holding on to some tension. How are your ankles doing? Rock them gently back and forth, to help them let go. Even the places where you don't normally think of tension and tightness accumulating, like your shins. Just close your eyes, travel down there in your imagination, and consciously help the tightness to let go.

Use your breathing to help you, too, and linger around in an area until you feel it is quite relaxed. As you breathe in, take the breath to the tense place and as you breathe out, let the breath take the tension or tightness away.

Move up from the feet, through the shins and the calves, to the knees, to the thighs, to the pelvis and torso.

Start from your hands, wrists, up the arms to the shoulders, everywhere giving permission for the body to relax and let go. From the shoulders up to the neck, and then on up to the head. Yes, even the brain can be holding tension. Remember to keep breathing, and the breath will help you let it go. As you do this exercise, take your time to go really, really slowly. Be gentle with yourself, and when you feel that an adjustment in your position will help the body to relax, make the movements small and easy until you find just the right spot. It's easiest, and most relaxing, to do the exercise as you are lying on your back. A little later, we suggest some things you can do with pillows or with a rolled-up towel to make yourself even more comfortable. A pillow under the knees, for example, is very relaxing for the lower back. Your body is always grateful for the attention, and if you take your time and persuade it gently, it will slip easily into relaxation.

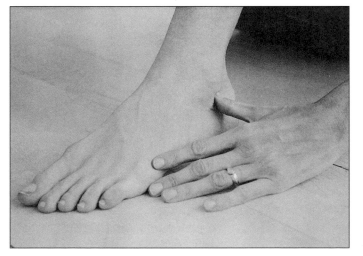

PICTURED ON THIS PAGE:
If you feel around below the ankle bone on the outside of the foot, you'll find a little hollow there. This is a point known in shiatsu as "calm sleep." If you apply pressure there, it will help to soothe and relax both body and mind so that the tossing and turning, the mental restlessness that can follow you even into your sleep, has a chance to settle down. This point is also good for back pain, hypertension and sciatica, restoring harmony to the body and helping you to have a "calm sleep."

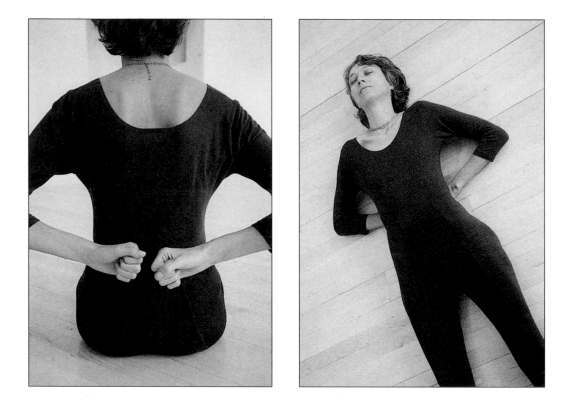

I F YOU DO the exercise pictured on this page first, it will help you to better be able to do the imagining task of the exercise pictured opposite. Both techniques relax and revitalize the kidneys, and in the process release a lot of holding and tension accumulated in the kidneys and lower back. The breath is used in these exercises too, as an aid in bringing your awareness to what you are doing and in helping the tension and holding to dissolve. Give yourself a few moments to relax and settle into the bed before actually beginning to do the techniques, so your breathing has a chance to settle and become natural.

PICTURED ON THIS PAGE:

M ake loose fists of your hands, and tuck them underneath the lower back where the kidneys are, as shown by our model here. If you have a firm mattress, this is fine to do on your bed – otherwise you might want to lie on a mat on the floor. Now, turn your attention to the area where your back meets the knuckles of your hands, and the feeling of pressure and relaxation as your breath rises and falls. Let your breath be relaxed and natural – no need to do any special breathing for this technique.

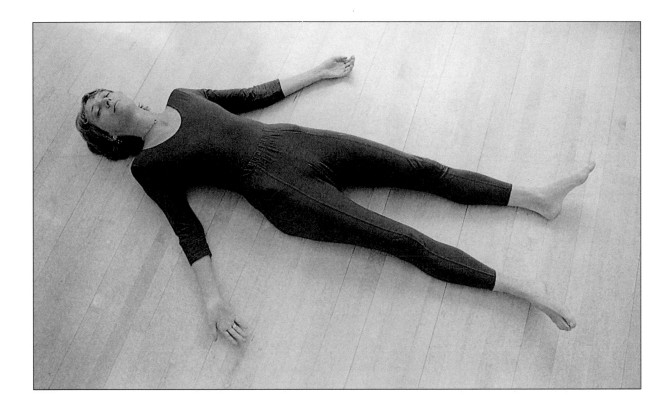

PICTURED AT RIGHT:

Most of the time when we lie on our backs, our breathing seems to be happening in the front of the body. This technique involves shifting this "normal" state of affairs and using our imaginations to let the back part of the body enjoy the relaxation and warmth that the breath brings with it.

Simply lie in a comfortable position on your back, giving yourself a few moments to settle into a relaxed and natural breathing pattern. Now, imagine that as your breath comes in, it is traveling along the spine, bathing the spine in light and warmth and relaxation. If the image doesn't come right away, be patient, and playful, and open to the "switch" – it will happen on its own, without needing you to "do" it.

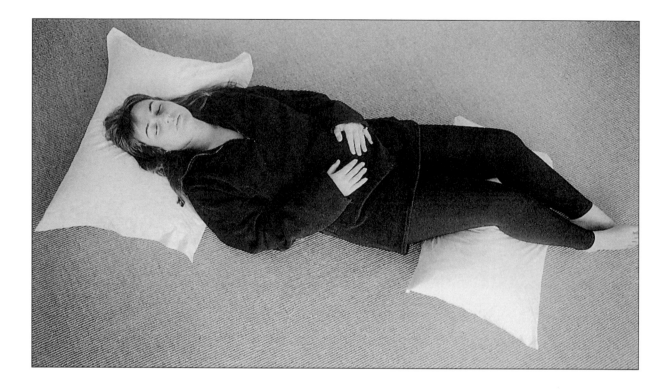

ONE THING WE haven't talked about yet is the condition of your bed – your body needs support, and you spend almost one third of your life in bed. So a good mattress is essential.

The other thing to consider is how many pillows you have available. Get lots! You can arrange them in all kinds of ways to give your body a feeling of being supported and comforted when it's feeling a bit battered and trying to protect itself.

Pillows under the knees can help relieve pain in the lower back. The sciatic pain that goes down the back of the leg from the buttocks can be eased by turning on your side, with your knees slightly bent, and putting a pillow between the knees. You can add a pillow or two behind your back, and create a delicious cocoon to curl up in after an especially hard day.

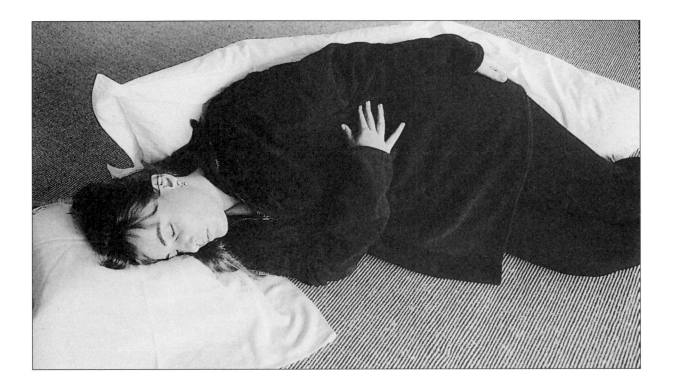

For people who gather a lot of tension in the neck and shoulders, a rolled-up towel is also very handy. Experiment until you get just the right thickness to place under your neck in place of a pillow – the right thickness is one that firmly supports the neck and still allows the head to lie flat on the mattress.

Just lie there, letting the head have the feeling of sinking, opening and relaxing the neck as the tension goes. You can combine this rolled-up towel device with the overall body relaxation technique described on page 146. Or, you can place a rolled up towel under your lower back instead of your fists to do the kidney-relaxation technique on page 148.

With the pillows, it's fine to experiment until you find arrangements that your body likes. If it helps you feel more comfortable and relaxed, it's good.... Sweet dreams!

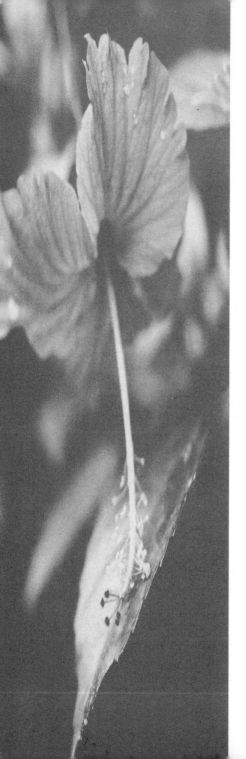

"If you accept the body in its absolute naturalness, it will help you tremendously. It will help your heart, nourish your heart. It will help your intelligence to become sharper, because the nourishment for the intellect comes from the body. Nourishment to the heart comes from the body. And if your head, your heart and your body are all in a symphony, then to find your being is the easiest thing in the world. But because they are in conflict, your whole life goes on being wasted in that conflict, conflict between instinct and intellect and intuition.

A wise man is one who creates a harmony between head, heart, and body. In this harmony one comes to the revelation of the source of one's life, the very centre, the soul. And that is the greatest ecstasy possible — not only to human beings but in this whole universe, nothing more is possible."[38]

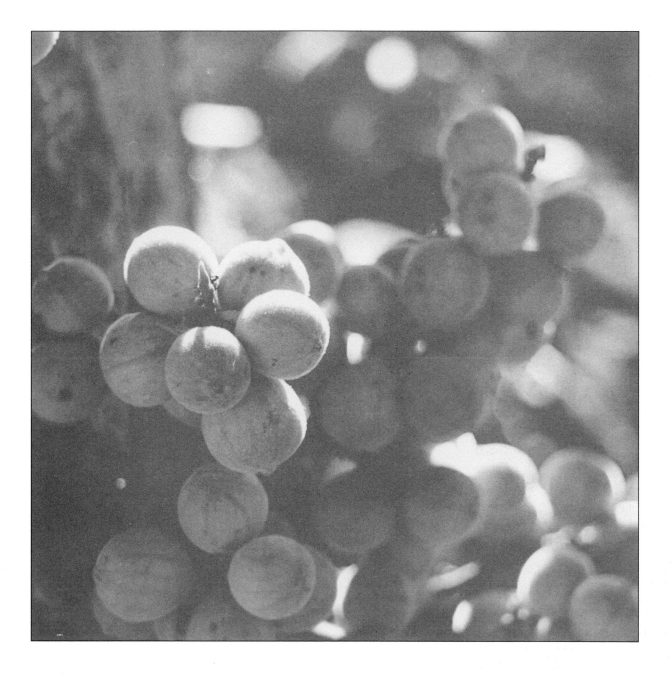

All footnoted quotations in this book have been taken from the published and unpublished talks of Osho, a 20th century enlightened mystic.

Osho taught philosophy at the University of Jabalpur before establishing the commune in Poona, India, which has become famous all over the world as a mecca for seekers wanting to experience meditation and transformation. His teachings have inspired millions of people of all ages and from all walks of life. He has been described by *The Sunday Times* as one of the 1000 Makers of the 20th Century, and by the *Sunday Mid-Day* (India) as one of the ten people - along with Gandhi, Nehru and Buddha - who have changed the destiny of India.

SOURCES

1 *From Unconsciousness to Consciousness*, chapter 29
2 *Ecstasy - The Forgotten Language*, chapter 7
3 *Ancient Music in the Pines*, chapter 3
4 *Ecstasy - The Forgotten Language*, chapter 7
5 *Hallelujah!*, chapter 31
6 *The Buddha: The Emptiness of the Heart*, chapter 3
7 *Dang Dang Doko Dang*, chapter 3
8 *Come Follow To You, Vol 2*, chapter 10
9 *Vigyan Bhairav Tantra, Vol 2*, chapter 15
10 *That Art Thou*, chapter 44
11 *The Razor's Edge*, chapter 21
12 *When the Shoe Fits*, chapter 1
13 *Nansen: The Point of Departure*, chapter 10
14 *The Further Shore*, chapter 2
15 *The Cypress in the Courtyard*, chapter 23
16 *The Madman's Guide to Enlightenment*, chapter 17
17 *Dance Your Way to God*, chapter 24
18 *The Empty Boat*, chapter 4
19 *Vigyan Bhairav Tantra, Vol 2*, chapter 23
20 *Early Talks*, chapter 4

21 *The Grass Grows By Itself*, chapter 1
22 *And The Flowers Showered*, chapter 3
23 *Vigyan Bhairav Tantra, Vol 1*, chapter 37
24 *The Hidden Splendor*, chapter 15
25 *From Unconsciousness to Consciousness*, chapter 1
26 *Take It Easy, Vol 2*, chapter 12
27 *I Am The Gate*, chapter 5
28 *Vedanta: Seven Steps to Samadhi*, chapter 12
29 *Vigyan Bhairav Tantra, Vol 1*, chapter 13
30 *The Secret of Secrets, Vol 1*, chapter 7
31 *Beloved of My Heart*, chapter 8
32 *When the Shoe Fits*, chapter 10
33 *The First Principle*, chapter 5
34 *Zarathustra: The Laughing Prophet*, chapter 13
35 *Turn On, Tune In and Drop the Lot*, chapter 24
36 *Just Like That*, chapter 7
37 *Only Losers Can Win in This Game*, chapter 16
38 *The Hidden Splendor*, chapter 25

FURTHER READING

We are pleased to recommend the following titles for those interested in further exploration some of the concepts and systems introduced in *BodyWisdom*.

DeLong Miller, Roberta: *Psychic Massage*, Harper San Francisco, 1975
Kunz, Kevin and Barbara: *Hand and Foot Reflexology*, 1986
Lundberg, Paul: *The Book of Shiatsu*, 1992
Masunaga, Shizuto with Wataru Ohashi: *Zen Shiatsu*, 1977
Namikashi, Toru: *The Complete Book of Shiatsu Therapy*, 1981
Osho: *Contemplation Before Sleep*, Boxtree, 1995
Osho: *Meditation, The First and Last Freedom*, Boxtree, 1985
Osho: *Morning Contemplation*, Boxtree, 1995
Osho: *Tantra: The Supreme Understanding*, The Rebel Publishing House, 1984
Teeguarden, Iona: *Accupressure Way of Health*, 1978
Van Lysebeth, Andre: *Yoga Self-Taught*, 1968
Yamamoto, Shizuko: *Barefoot Shiatsu*, 1979

The following German-language titles are also recommended:

Bordella, David: *Befreite Lebensenergie*, 1978
deLangre, Jacques: *Do-In 2*, 1978

OSHO COMMUNE INTERNATIONAL

The Osho Commune International in Poona, India, guided by Osho's vision might be described as a laboratory, an experiment in creating the "New Man" — a human being who lives in harmony with himself and his environment, and who is free from all ideologies and belief systems which now divide humanity.

The Commune's Osho Multiversity offers numerous workshops, groups and trainings, presented by its nine different faculties. These are attended by thousands of visitors from around the world every year.

All these programmes are designed to help people to find the knack of meditation: the passive witnessing of thoughts, emotions, and actions, without judgement or identification. Unlike many traditional Eastern disciplines, meditation at Osho Commune is an inseparable part of everyday life - working, relating or just being. The result is that people do not renounce the world but bring to it a spirit of awareness and celebration, in a deep reverence for life.

The highlight of the day at the Commune is the meeting of the Osho White Robe Brotherhood. This two-hour celebration of music, dance and silence, with a discourse from Osho, is unique — a complete meditation in itself where thousands of seekers, in Osho's words, "dissolve into a sea of consciousness."

FOR FURTHER INFORMATION

Many of Osho's books have been translated and published in a variety of languages worldwide. For information about Osho, his meditations, books, tapes, and the address of an Osho meditation/information centre near you, contact:

Osho International Foundation
24 St James's Street
London SW1A 1HA, UK

Osho Commune International
17 Koregaon Park
Poona 411001, India

ABOUT THE AUTHORS

Anando Würzburger studied massage at the Esalen Foundation in California and practiced Hatha Yoga in the early 1970s. She has been a disciple of the Indian mystic Osho since 1978. Trained in Eastern healing concepts at the Osho International Academy of Healing Arts, Anando is also a therapist in rebirthing and bioenergetics, and has worked in Germany as a Shiatsu practitioner and therapist since 1982. At the Osho Commune International in Poona, India, she developed the Osho Hara Awareness Massage, and designed the Hara Training in centering, grounding, and healing, which is offered by the Commune several times a year. When she is not conducting trainings and offering sessions in Poona, Anando lives in Cologne, Germany.

Amiyo Ruhnke is a former advertising art director who now divides her time between London, New York, and Poona, India. She has been a disciple of the Indian mystic Osho since 1981, and has practiced meditation since that time. Her interest in exploring the bodymind connection arose when she took up the study of the Japanese martial art Aikido.